the clever guts diet recipe book

The information contained in this book is provided for general purposes only. It is not intended as, and should not be relied upon as, medical advice. The publisher and authors are not responsible for any specific health needs that may require medical supervision. If you have underlying health problems, or have any doubts about the advice contained in this book, you should contact a qualified medical, dietary or appropriate professional.

Clare Bailey has asserted her right under the Copyright, Designs and Patents Act 1988 to be identified as the author of this work. All rights reserved. No part of this publication may be reproduced, stored in a retrieval system or transmitted in any form, or by any means (electronic, mechanical, or otherwise) without the prior written permission of both the copyright owners and the publisher.

A CIP catalogue record for this book
is available from the British Library.

Published in 2017 by Short Books
Unit 316
ScreenWorks,
22 Highbury Grove
N5 2ER

10 9 8 7 6 5 4 3 2 1

Copyright © Parenting Matters Ltd
Photographs copyright © Joe Sarah
Food styling: Dara Sutin
Design by Andrew Smith

Printed in Italy by L.E.G.O SpA

the clever guts diet

recipe book

150 delicious recipes to mend your gut
and boost your health and wellbeing

Dr Clare Bailey WITH
nutritionist Joy Skipper

PHOTOGRAPHY BY JOE SARAH

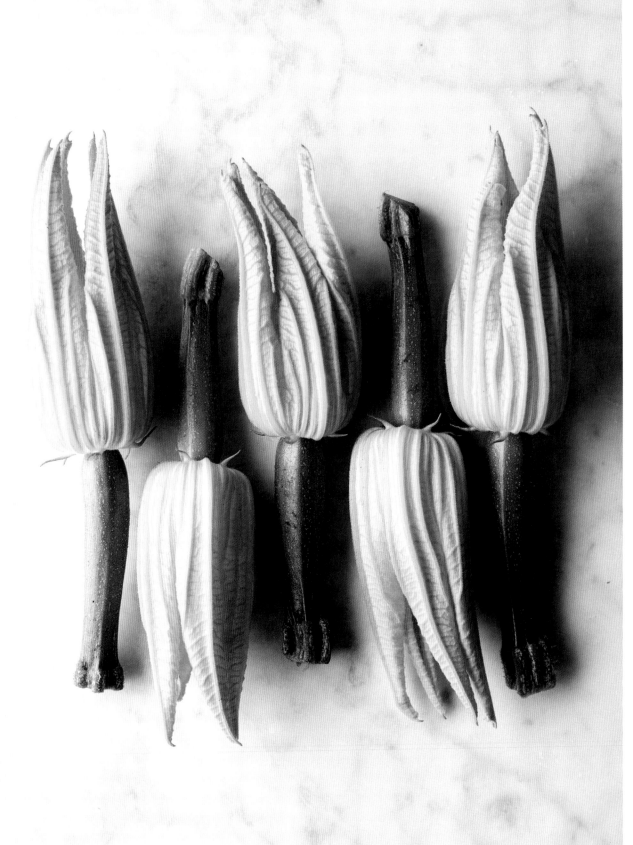

Contents

Foreword by Dr Michael Mosley .... page 6

Introduction by Dr Clare Bailey .... page 8

The Clever Guts Diet .... page 10

1 Breakfast .... page 30

2 Light Meals, Soups and Salads .... page 52

3 Dressings and Flavourings .... page 114

4 Main Dishes .... page 124

5 Clever Veg .... page 158

6 Ferments .... page 178

7 Treats .... page 192

Meal Planners .... page 214

Index .... page 218

Foreword by Dr Michael Mosley

Hippocrates, the father of modern medicine, claimed over 2000 years ago that 'all diseases begin in the gut'. It's taken a long time, but we are beginning to realise just how profound Hippocrates' insight really was. There's never been as much interest in the human gut and its tiny inhabitants, the trillions of microbes that make up the microbiome, as there is now. New research tools have enabled scientists to probe the previously secret world of the gut, and uncover more and more about the impact that the 1000 different species that live down there have on you, and you have on them. Thanks to advances in DNA technology we have learnt more surprising things about the gut in the last few years than in all of previous human history. It's been a bit like Galileo inventing the telescope and using it to discover a whole new universe, one that is larger and more complex than anything that earlier generations could ever have imagined.

These new discoveries about the gut are not just of academic interest. It is becoming ever clearer just how important the microbiome is for keeping the rest of our body, and brain, in good shape. We have recently learnt, for example, that the mix of microbes in our gut can strongly influence our weight, our mood and even our immune system. The tragedy is that a modern diet, which relies heavily on processed food, along with the widespread over-use of antibiotics, has laid waste to the modern microbiome. This helps explain some of the dramatic increases we've seen over the last few decades in obesity, type 2 diabetes, allergic diseases and food intolerances.

What's the link? Well, an addiction to junk food and the indiscriminate use of antibiotics have helped devastate our 'Old Friends'. These are the microbes that live in our guts and which evolved with us. They are essential to our health. Devastating these Old Friends has in turn made space for unhealthy microbes to flourish, those that encourage inflammation, weight gain and, possibly, depression.

The good news is that it's never too late to do something to help those Old Friends recover. Adding new foods to your diet, doing a bit more exercise, simply getting outdoors more, can all have a positive impact on your gut health.

This book is only possible because of the extraordinary work done by scientists from many different countries, who have generously shared their time and research. But it is also a labour of love by its main author, Dr Clare Bailey. I have known Clare for over 35 years. We met on our first day at medical school and married soon after graduating. As well as being a dedicated doctor, Clare has always been passionate and adventurous about food. When she was working with the Save the Children Fund in a remote part of the Amazon jungle, she was fascinated as much by her medical work there as by the unusual foods they were eating. This included, on one occasion, a giant toad, 'as large as a chicken', which they shared between four of them. Apparently it was delicious.

These days Clare is a busy GP who, amongst other things, uses her love of food and interest in nutrition to help her patients improve their blood sugar levels and reverse their type 2 diabetes by losing weight, rather than relying on medication. This led to her writing the bestselling *8-Week Blood Sugar Diet Recipe Book*.

Building on what she has learnt, she is now using food to improve her patients' gut health as well as their gut size. The recipes in this book are the product of the latest science. They are gut-friendly, but taste, flavour and simplicity are equally important. They are also written with a busy person in mind, so the ingredients should be easy to access and inexpensive.

I have greatly enjoyed eating my way through the recipes in this book and I hope you do too.

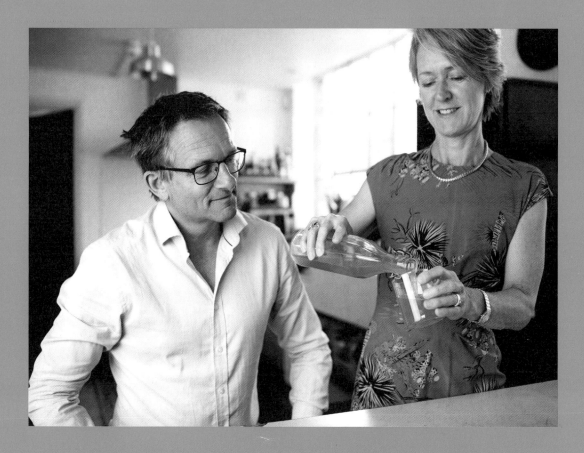

Introduction by Dr Clare Bailey

I have been working as a doctor for over 30 years and in that time have seen a lot of remarkable medical changes and innovations, but to discover a whole new world, a new organ, if you like, one that produces chemicals, controls our appetites, moods and metabolism, that can work for us or against us depending on how we treat it… this really is a new frontier. We are starting to discover this new world's many inhabitants, and to learn what they do, what disturbs them and how they can be nurtured or defeated. Welcome to the microbiome, the trillions of microbes that live in your intestines.

This book will introduce you to some of these tiny guys busily working away to keep you happy and healthy. More importantly, it will show you how you can help them help you; how you can feed them the variety of fibre and nutrients they need and top them up with probiotics, the healthy microbes found in fermented foods.

In recent decades, we have abandoned traditional ways of eating, relying on instant and processed foods, which more often than not are high in sugars. The average adult eats some 200 sandwiches a year, and the most common choice of filling is cheese, followed closely by ham. A limited diet of this nature is bound to have a negative impact on our health and particularly on our gut health. Nor is it enough to live on a 'healthy' diet of avocados, sweet potatoes, bagged spinach and cherry tomatoes and think you've got it sorted…

Like us, our microbiome thrives on variety, which is why the recipes here offer a diverse range of proteins, whether plant-based, seafood or meat. It is why we encourage you to eat veg of every colour and try new foods and flavours.

You may be reading this book because you have trouble with your gut. Perhaps you suspect a food intolerance or that you have Irritable Bowel Syndrome (IBS), and feel that your gut is in need of a reboot (see page 24). Or maybe you are doing this simply to broaden your horizons and improve your diet with some gut-friendly recipes – in which case try as many as you can. This is not a diet focused on weight loss, though this can happen as part of the process, particularly if you incorporate the 5:2 approach (see page 18).

As someone who loves experimenting with food, I hope most of all that you enjoy the meals we have put together and that they make you feel well and content with life.

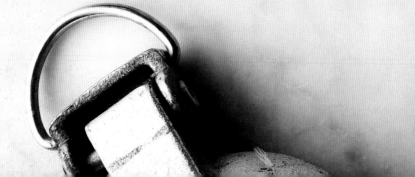

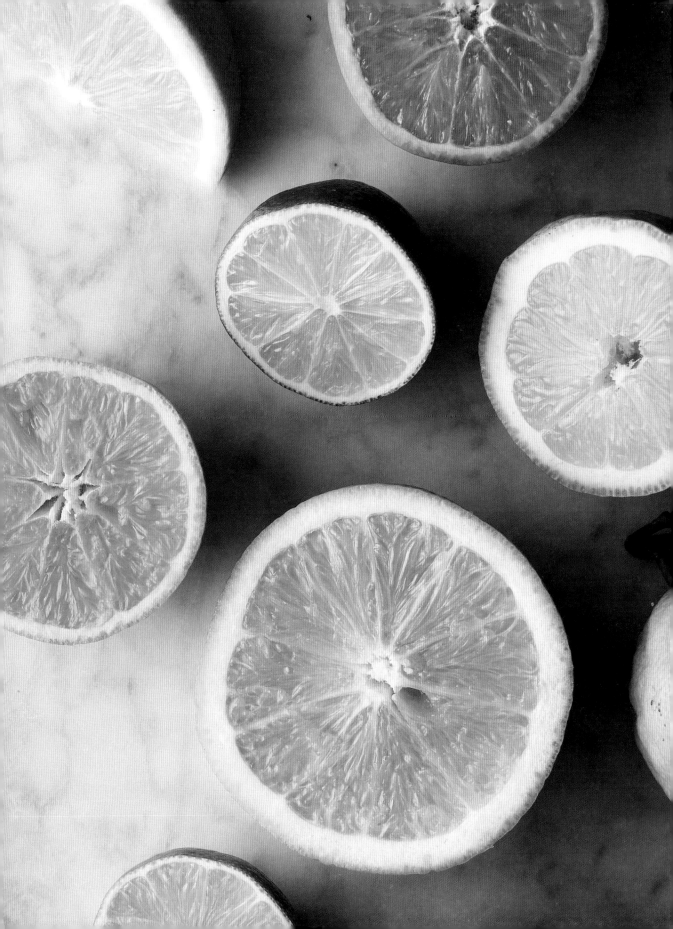

The Clever Guts Diet

Based on the Mediterranean way of eating

This diet is based on 'real food' – plenty of vegetables, fruits, nuts, beans, olive oil, cheese, meat and oily fish, but relatively little starchy pizza, pasta, potato or bread. We call it 'Mediterranean style' because although many of the recipes have a Mediterranean twist, the recipes draw on healthy cuisines from all over the world. Most of the ingredients you will be familiar with; some (such as fermented foods and seaweed) will be more surprising. Where it is convenient we go back to more traditional ways of preparation that may have been lost in the era of fast, processed and packaged foods. That said, none of the recipes are particularly complicated or time-consuming. The emphasis is on freshness, good flavours and being 'doable'. I have plenty of patients who don't particularly like to cook and I keep them in mind when I am creating recipes. We recommend using natural single ingredients where possible: that way you know what is in your food and don't have to decipher the secret code words of a dozen or more added ingredients.

We love this diet because as well as being incredibly tasty, it is the best researched on the planet. Big studies have shown that compared to a diet that is low in fat and high in starchy carbs, this form of Mediterranean diet – based on eating fairly low Glycaemic Index (GI) foods which tend to be higher in fibre and release sugars more slowly – will help you keep the weight off, halve your risk of developing type 2 diabetes, reduce your risk of developing cancer (particularly breast cancer) and keep your brain in good shape. Last but by no means least, it will help you maintain a healthy microbiome.

Low in sugars and starchy carbohydrates

Eating lots of white carbs and sugary, processed foods will not only damage your waistline, but your microbiome as well. These foods will encourage the growth of unhealthy microbes, which in turn cause inflammation.

The problem is that sugars and starchy carbs are everywhere, not just in the obvious items like fizzy drinks, biscuits and donuts. They are in pretty much every processed food you buy – often listed as separate ingredients, such as glucose, maltose syrup, maltodextrin, dextrose, fruit juice concentrates, corn fructose, high fructose corn syrup, malt syrup, raw sugar, lactose, cane sugar… There are over 60 different names that may appear on food labels, most of them sounding fairly innocuous. Another reason to avoid processed foods if you can.

Retrain your palate and your microbiome by cutting back on sugar. Believe it or not, as your gut biome changes, the cravings will fade. Feeding up the good microbes with a healthy diet will gradually silence the messages being sent out by the sugar-loving ones that are calling for more. You should notice a difference within a few weeks.

Skip the sweeteners too – these cheat your system into expecting a sugar fix and help maintain your sweet tooth (they're often many times sweeter-tasting than the real stuff). They can also damage a healthy microbiome. Kick the habit and your tastes will change. You will become more sensitive to other flavours and enjoy much lower levels of sugar, or even start finding it cloying and slightly sickly. (See chapter 7 for low-sugar treats.)

Choose more vegetables – try and ensure they take up at least half a plate. Make them interesting and varied. Add butter or olive oil. Pep them up with flavouring such as chilli flakes, cumin or a squeeze of lemon. Stir-fry your greens. Add garlic. If you are not a great fan of veg, start your meal with them, so that you are eating them when you are hungry. They may become your favourite part of the meal. Michael used to shuffle his veg around his plate with little interest. He now even adds extra – and consumes far fewer starchy carbs as a result. (See chapter 5 for veg dishes.)

Get your digestive juices going with a light, enzyme-inducing salad at the beginning of your meal to improve your digestion (see page 55).

Focused on good food not calories

We have included calories as an aid, not as a focus. The main reason they are recorded is to help those who are including a 5:2 intermittent fasting element in their diet (see page 18) as this has been shown to improve gut health as well as increase weight loss and boost the metabolism. The calories are recorded per portion unless otherwise stated. They are also rounded to the nearest zero. Don't get too caught up on them. Whatever the calorie content of the food you put in your mouth, the mix of microbes in your gut will help decide what proportion of it is absorbed. Some people have much more calorie-rich poo than others. Different foods behave differently, depending on how you prepare them and what you eat them with. So, for example, eating a baked potato is likely to raise your blood sugars less if you add butter or cheese. Who would have guessed?

Food Groups and the Microbiome

Protein

As protein cannot be stored, the average adult needs to eat around 45-60g of it a day. However, unless you are doing a very physical job or extreme amounts of exercise, more is not necessarily better. This is a moderate-protein diet, not a high-protein diet.

Variety is all when it comes to gut health, so eat as broad a range of protein as you can. Quality proteins include meat, oily fish, eggs, seafood, tofu and cheese. Other good sources include soya (edamame) beans, Quorn, nuts and tempeh. There are strong ethical reasons why you might want to avoid meat, but it is undoubtedly an excellent source of protein and important nutrients such as iron. We recommend eating outdoor-reared meat if possible. Eat less, but better quality – ideally red meat no more than twice a week. It is advised to restrict processed meats (such as salami and bacon) as they are more likely to contain additives, preservatives or hydrogenated oils.

Healthy natural fats

These are found in plant foods, such as nuts, seeds, olive oil and avocado, and in dairy products, as well as meat and seafood – oily fish being one of the best sources. Increasing the proportion of healthy fats you eat helps to reset your metabolism and reduce blood sugars. Fat slows the release of starchy carbohydrates and sugars (hence the baked potato conundrum above). Being slow to burn, it provides a steady source of energy that doesn't stimulate the release of insulin (the fat storage hormone). That said, there are oils that you should try to avoid – the trans and partially hydrogenated fats that are mainly present in spreads and processed foods, such as biscuits and pastries.

Dairy

Foods such as yoghurt and cheese are an excellent source of calcium and protein, and are not the demons responsible for increasing the risk of developing heart disease or type 2 diabetes that we once thought they were. However, dairy products contain the sugar lactose, which can cause digestive symptoms, such as bloating, cramps and diarrhoea. Around 75% of the world's population are lactose-intolerant, and if you have it mildly you may not have identified it as the cause of your symptoms. If this is the case, it may be worth trying a brief exclusion diet to see if it helps (as described in Phase1 – see page 25). We do include dairy products in many of the recipes, but suggest alternatives, such as nut or soy products, wherever possible.

Grains

We are not anti-grain by any means; in fact, whole grains are found to be beneficial. But because many grains contain gluten which can irritate the gut, and in some people cause problems, we have tried to minimise using it in our recipes. We have used traditional, lower-gluten grains, such as rye or spelt, or 'artisan' bread-making techniques such as sourdough, where the fermentation process breaks down much of the gluten, making it easier to tolerate.

For those who are avoiding gluten altogether, many gluten-free flours are now available. They are made with a blend of ingredients, such as rice flour, potato flour, tapioca, maize and buckwheat, and are designed for baking. However, they are often white and highly refined, and tend to lack the healthy fibre needed by your microbiome. We would urge you where possible to use wholegrain alternatives such as buckwheat flour, which, despite the misleading name, is gluten-free, or wholemeal chickpea flour, also known as gram flour or besan, or indeed nut flours or ground almonds, which are also high in protein and healthy natural oils. There are lots of tricks to help produce a bread-like texture or softer cakes, such as adding xanthum gum.

Fibre

Fibre acts like a broom for the digestive system, helping the gut to push waste through the intestine. It is broadly made up of non-digestible carbohydrates and acts as a source of energy and nutrients for the creatures that live in your gut. We should all be aiming to eat at least 35g of fibre a day; unfortunately, the average Western diet contains less than half of that.

Most foods contain a mix of soluble and insoluble fibre. Soluble fibre attracts water and partially dissolves, forming a thick gel which helps to create the stool and move it through the intestines. It can also help reduce heart disease. Soluble fibre is found in foods like oatmeal, barley, lentils, beans, potatoes, carrots, bananas, avocados and okra.

Insoluble fibre doesn't dissolve; it is more 'scratchy' and adds bulk to the stool. Two of the most important types of it, as far as your gut is concerned, are inulin and fructooligosacharides. These are prebiotics, which are not digested in the small intestine, but continue on down the gut to become an important source of nutrients for the microbiome, promoting the growth of beneficial bacteria. These bacteria, through fermentation of fibre in the colon, produce the vital short-chain fatty acids, such as butyrate, proprionate and acetate, which in turn play an important role in health and disease. Fructooligosacharides are also a natural sweetener.

Insoluble fibre is found in foods such as asparagus, chicory, Jerusalem artichokes, onions, stringy beans, wheat bran, celery and tough stems of cabbage or kale. In some people it can exacerbate symptoms of IBS, so we include less of this in Phase 1 recipes.

Prebiotics and probiotics

Prebiotics are non-digestible carbohydrates, usually fibre, as we saw above, that have beneficial effects, particularly through encouraging the growth of gut-friendly micro-organisms. They are like the fertiliser that helps the grass grow in a lawn.

Probiotics are like the seeds that you scatter on the lawn to keep it lush and compete with the weeds. They are 'friendly' live bacteria, found naturally in fermented foods such as sauerkraut, kefir and yoghurt (see chapter 6), which work in a variety of ways along the digestive tract, boosting healthy microbes and driving down numbers of the harmful ones. We love them!

Polyphenols and phytonutrients

Polyphenols are the most common antioxidants in our food and tend to be found in plant fibre. They have anti-inflammatory properties and are good for your gut health as well as for your brain and heart. As much as 90-95% of the polyphenol-rich foods you take in make it down to the colon, where they are processed by microbes and encourage the growth of beneficial bacteria. Herbs, spices, nuts, seeds, berries, teas, red wine and dark chocolate contain high quantities of polyphenols, and we have included many of these in our recipes.

Phytonutrients are natural components of plants that keep them healthy, protecting them from disease and damage. Their antioxidant and anti-inflammatory properties also provide significant health benefits and help to preserve a healthy microbial balance in the gut. Phytonutrients are concentrated in the pigments in the skin of fruit and vegetables, so the key is to eat a wide variety of colours – aim for two or more of each per day.

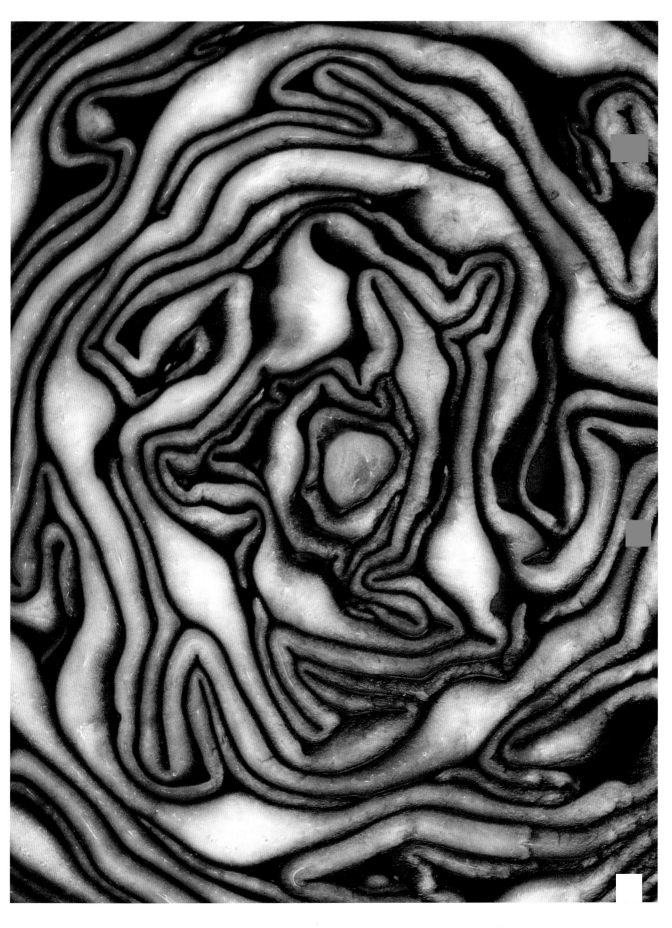

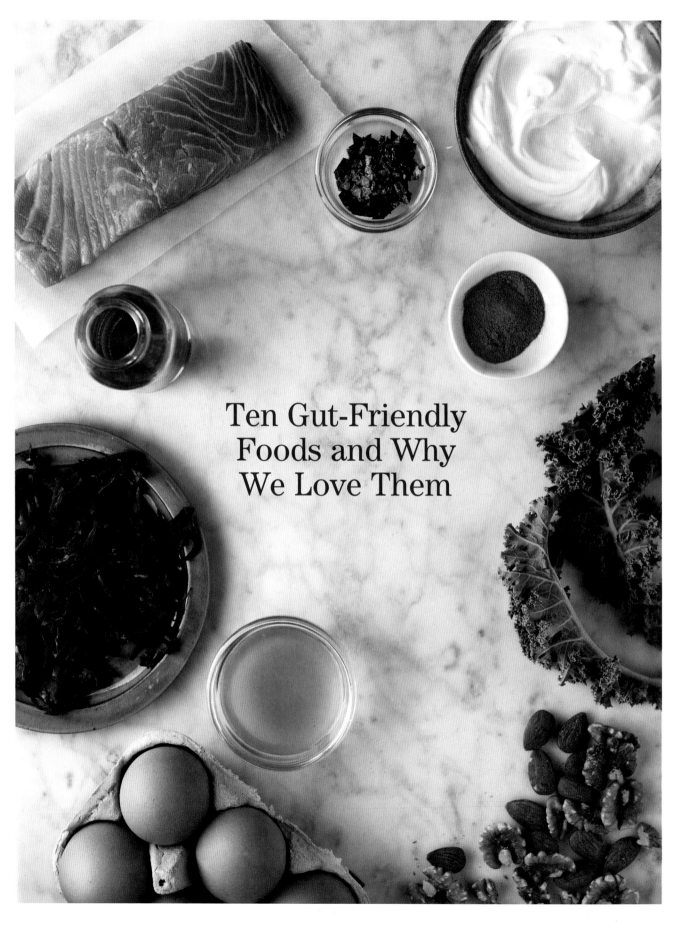

Ten Gut-Friendly
Foods and Why
We Love Them

1. **Olive oil**. As well as adding flavour and taste – and being safe to cook with – olive oil is one of the healthiest fats you can eat, rich in a range of polyphenols and antioxidants which are good at damping down inflammation.

2. **Oily fish.** Like olive oil, oily fish is full of good fats. The key ingredient is omega 3. Unfortunately, white fish, like cod, don't contain many omega 3 fatty acids and don't provide the same health benefits.

3. **Nuts**. Nuts have had a bad rap because they are oily and high in calories. However, there is very good evidence that the odd handful of nuts, eaten as a snack, will cut your risk of heart disease. They are also high in protein and fibre, and satiating.

4. **Full-fat live Greek-style yoghurt**. Not only tasty and filling, this form of yoghurt is also rich in health-inducing bacteria like *Lactobacillus*. The evidence that full-fat is better for you than low-fat is compelling. Plenty of studies have found that regularly eating full-fat yoghurt leads to less weight gain and a lower risk of diseases such as type 2 diabetes.

5. **Vegetables and fruit**. Everyone knows that fruit and veg are good for us, but even those who eat their five a day tend to stick to a very limited range. And that means our microbiome ends up being pretty limited as well. A simple solution is to add more colour to your plate...

6. **Eggs.** Not so long ago we were warned not to eat more than a couple of eggs a week, yet it turns out that the fear of cholesterol in eggs was totally misplaced. Eggs are a superb source of protein, rich in vitamins and minerals.

7. **Fermented foods**. Fermentation occurs when microbes in the food convert sugars into other compounds. The unique flavours and textures in them are due to the different species of bacteria and yeasts. Wine, cheese, yoghurt and chocolate are all fermented foods, as are kimchi, sauerkraut, kefir, kombucha, pickles and miso. The microbes in fermented foods are also far more likely than most other bacteria to make it safely down into your colon because they are extremely resistant to acid, having been reared in an acidic environment.

8. **Turmeric**. Turmeric contains at least 200 different compounds, but the one that's of particular interest to scientists is called curcumin. Evidence shows that turmeric has powerful antioxidant and anti-inflammatory properties, is good at inhibiting the growth of 'bad' bacteria, and fungi, and indirectly protects the wall of the intestine.

9. **Live apple cider vinegar.** This is another fermented food that is now hugely popular. A shot of apple cider vinegar taken before breakfast reduces blood sugar levels and there is evidence that it can also reduce cholesterol.

10. **Seaweed.** Seaweed is rich in fibre, packed with nutrients and has been shown to lead to a significant reduction in inflammation and an increase in insulin sensitivity.

Intermittent Fasting and Gut Health

We now know that intermittent fasting – short periods of reducing your calorie intake – improves your metabolic markers beyond those expected for weight loss. It also reduces blood sugars, leads to improvements in the lining of the gut and boosts the health of the microbiome. Giving your gut a rest from having to constantly digest food allows the lining to regenerate and encourages the growth of good bacteria like *Akkermansia*.

There are various different ways of practising intermittent fasting – from simply increasing your overnight fast to 12-14 hours, to doing prolonged periods of 800-calorie fasting as Michael outlines in the *8-Week Blood Sugar Diet*, or the popular 5:2 fasting approach that he sets out in *The Fast Diet* (5 days eating normally, 2 days on 500-600 calories).

We have included many recipes for those of you who are intermittent fasting – with an updated regimen of 800-calorie fast days. If you like the look of the higher-calorie recipes, but want to lose weight, we would recommend on fast days having half the stated portion and adding more vegetables.

Simply avoiding snacks is the minimum 'fasting' you could do. Most snacks prevent your body from going into fat-burning mode and cheat your microbiome of the chance to repair the gut lining between meals. If you must snack, choose unsalted, unflavoured nuts. Or snack on chopped veg or even a small amount of dark chocolate (at least 70% cocoa solids).

Tips for your 800-calorie 5:2 fasting days:

- **Plan fasting days** in advance.

- **Make sure you increase your water intake** as you miss out on the fluids in your usual food and you lose water when you burn fat. Aim for 2-3 litres a day.

- **Soups are surprisingly satiating, cheap and practical.** They are also more slowly digested. You can take them to work for lunch and keep portions in the freezer. Go for the non-starchy vegetable or clear broths like Quick Seaweed Miso Soup (page 61).

- **Drinking hot drinks suppresses appetite:** teas, coffee or Turmeric Tea (see page 21).

- **Use flavour enhancers** so each meal is as tasty as possible, for example lemon, pepper, lime, chilli, garlic, gherkins, mustard, herbs. They add very little in terms of calories.

- **Monitor blood sugars regularly if you are diabetic:** ideally twice daily at different times of the day at first. Consult your doctor before you begin the diet.

- **Side effects:** tiredness, lightheadedness and headaches (these are often related to dehydration), hunger (this comes in waves and passes so try to 'surf the wave') and feeling colder. All of these should settle over a week or so and are usually less noticeable if you increase the amount of fat you eat in your diet.

- **Avoid fasting or discuss with your doctor first if:** your BMI is below 20, you have a history of eating disorders, are under 18 years of age, on medication, are pregnant or breastfeeding, have a significant psychiatric disorder, are unwell or have a significant medical condition, are recovering from surgery, are frail or have other medical conditions.

The first few weeks can be tough, but your body adapts. Your appetite settles. In fact most people feel better and find they have more energy and a clearer head. It helps to get support. The website thebloodsugardiet.com provides plenty of useful resources and the opportunity to join a supportive, well-informed community.

Establishing Healthy Habits

Try to use this book to build healthy habits, whether you are hoping to improve your gut health and digestion or simply wanting to feel your best. One of the most important things you can do, right at the start, is involve other people. Tell your friends and family what you're planning and what you hope to achieve. Try to persuade one of them to join you, as being part of something bigger means you are more likely to succeed. Join an online community (such as cleverguts.com) for advice and support.

If, despite your best intentions, you find you are struggling, question your excuses. What is getting in the way? It can be uncomfortable making changes but stick with it and your better habits will become automatic.

Plan ahead – this helps to bypass 'willpower', which is usually in short supply and easily gets used up. Practise a bit of kitchen hygiene – remove temptations from your surfaces and cupboards. Research has shown that households with cereal packets or biscuits on view are more likely to be overweight than those who keep them in the cupboards, out of sight.

If you are watching your weight, practise portion control. Use a smaller plate, eat slowly and listen to your appetite. This will give your body time to send the message that you are full. If you have raised blood sugars, these vital feedback loops stop working, leaving you constantly hungry and unsatisfied. It's not greed, just the system out of kilter. If you stick with it, your blood sugars should improve and the normal feedback system will re-establish itself, leaving you feeling comfortably full after eating. My patients often say that after the first week or two it gets much easier.

Get up a bit earlier – 10 more minutes gives you time to make a healthy swap from toast and jam or processed cereals to a delicious and filling breakfast, such as scrambled eggs or porridge (see chapter 1 for more breakfast suggestions).

Get to bed earlier – better sleep enhances concentration, resets your stress levels, improves your metabolism and has a beneficial effect on your microbiome. Aim for 7-8 hours' sleep most days. Consider taking sleep-inducing inulin powder before bed to help your gut to help you sleep (go to cleverguts.com for more information).

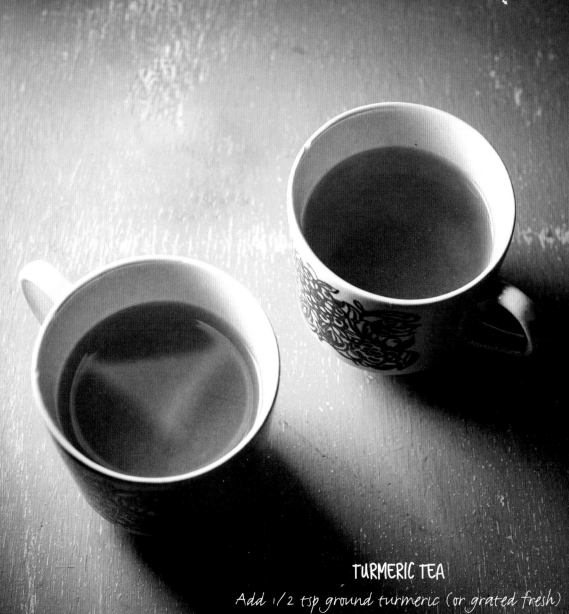

TURMERIC TEA

Add 1/2 tsp ground turmeric (or grated fresh)
to a cup of hot water, with 1/2 tsp cinnamon
and a squeeze of lemon, for a light, nutritious
drink or a tangy, aromatic digestif to be
sipped after a meal. Just remember to keep
stirring the brew as some of the spices slowly
sink to the bottom of the cup.

Reduce stress – easier said than done, but we know that chronic pressure and anxiety wreak havoc on your stress hormones, mood and immune system. The stress hormone cortisol, for example, increases blood sugars and promotes the storage of unhealthy abdominal fat. These hormones are also likely to have an adverse effect on your metabolism, eating patterns, gut bacteria and, most importantly, on how you feel in yourself. A vicious cycle of low mood, less motivation and comfort eating may follow. Try to accept things you can't change and deal with things you can. Make some changes, even small ones (though perhaps not all at once!). Mindfulness is an excellent evidence-based way to de-stress and to reduce rumination and the tendency to get stuck in a loop, preoccupied with seemingly insoluble issues.

Practise mindful eating – sit down at a table to eat, and be present in the moment so you are able to focus on what you are eating, to taste it, to savour it. Become aware of the flavour and texture. Is it slightly bitter? Can you taste sweetness or a hint of sour? Or both? Celebrate and enjoy your food. The more interesting and varied, the better for both you and your microbiome. By contrast, if you eat in front of the TV, you probably won't notice any of these satisfying experiences and are likely to eat more in the process. Having your meal at a table can be helpful in other ways too, particularly if you are eating with others. It can lift your mood and keep you connected. But don't let others push you to eat more than you want, even if it is done as a demonstration of love – learn to say no pleasantly and mean it.

Get more active – we all know that doing exercise is fantastically good for us. It boosts our mood, helps us sleep, cuts our risk of almost every chronic disease (from cancer to dementia) and burns a few calories. There is now good evidence that regular exercise will also improve the quality and diversity of your microbiome. Ideally you should do a mix of exercises that build muscle strength and aerobic fitness.

To keep his muscles in shape Michael likes (well, perhaps not 'likes') to do a mix of press-ups, squats and sit-ups most morning. For his heart and lungs he takes the dog for the occasional run and cycles where he can, incorporating high-intensity bursts. I try to run for 20 minutes 3 times a week when I can, adding short high-intensity bursts up hills, as well as practise yoga (which incidentally has recently been found to improve gut health, too). The important thing is to push yourself so your heart rate goes up.

If you are not able to commit to specific exercises, you can do yourself a huge amount of good simply by getting outside and moving more. Get your hands dirty, whether in the garden or the park, to get more bugs in your life!

Before You Start

If you have any significant medical problems or very troublesome gut symptoms, we recommend you consult a health professional first. There may be medical reasons for your symptoms that need checking first, such as undiagnosed coeliac disease, which can cause low-grade symptoms or even no symptoms at all, but can still lead to significant complications. Other conditions such as inflammatory bowel disease may require further investigation or management. It is important to rule out other potentially significant causes of your symptoms before embarking on dietary changes. It may help to do the programme with professional support. If you are underweight, suspect you have a food allergy, have other significant medical problems or are frail or unwell, we would not advise embarking on this programme.

Seek urgent medical advice if you: are passing blood and/or mucus; have severe and/or persistent abdominal pain; experience unexplained, unplanned weight loss or loss of appetite; have a recent change in bowel habit; suffer from anaemia or a deficiency in important vitamins or nutrients; have persistent diarrhoea and/or vomiting.

Fortunately, food allergies are relatively uncommon. But if you suspect you have one, it is very important that you see your doctor and get tested as it could be life-threatening. Symptoms normally occur within minutes of being in contact with or eating the relevant substance. The typical reaction might involve a blotchy red rash, which is raised and itchy. There may be vomiting and/or severe gut symptoms such as diarrhoea; respiratory symptoms resulting in wheezing and difficulty breathing; itching or swelling of the lips, tongue and palate; or, very rarely, sudden collapse. Once your health professional has helped identify the food substance, you can take measures to avoid it and, if needed, keep emergency medication to hand. An allergy is different from a food intolerance, which is a non-allergic hypersensitivity, and is much more common. With an intolerance, the onset tends to be delayed by hours, not minutes, and the symptoms are more variable. If you find yourself excluding food, or food groups for a long period of time, we recommend that you consult a professional to ensure that the full clinical picture is considered and that you are getting a healthy balanced diet.

Rebooting Your Biome with Phases 1 and 2

Most people who pursue the Clever Guts diet will be doing so to benefit from its general health improvements – a happier, stronger gut and metabolism, as well as weight loss, a reduction in blood sugars and just feeling better in themselves. However, for those who have gut- and health-related issues that are possibly due to a food sensitivity or intolerance, we would suggest you also try Michael's 2-phase programme (see *The Clever Guts Diet*) to reboot your biome.

We would strongly advise that for at least three days beforehand you keep a food diary in which you record the foods eaten and your responses to them. This may come in useful if you decide to see a professional about your symptoms. To download our Clever Guts Daily Food and Symptoms Diary, go to cleverguts.com/reboot-your-biome/

A word on **FODMAPs** (Fermentable Oligosaccharides, Disaccharides, Monosaccharides and Polyols) – these are a group of poorly absorbed carbohydrates that are found in certain fruits and vegetables. In some people with gut problems, like IBS, these foods get fermented in the bowel, producing more gas, causing wind, bloating and distension. They can also draw extra fluid into the bowel causing diarrhoea. Although many of these substances are good for a healthy bowel and help feed the microbiome, they may need to be reduced or avoided in IBS and in Phase 1 of the programme. The Clever Guts Diet is not specifically a low FODMAP diet, but where possible we have highlighted foods that might exacerbate symptoms of IBS. See cleverguts.com for more information.

.... and **nightshade vegetables.** On our website, cleverguts.com, people sometimes ask if they should avoid this group of vegetables, of which there are many, including tomatoes, bell peppers, aubergines and potatoes. They are the edible parts of flowering plants that belong to the Solanaceae family, and are technically classified as fruit. Some people have found they feel better when they reduce their consumption of these foods or remove them completely on the basis that they may contribute to inflammation and leaky gut. If you suspect a problem, it may be worth excluding them for two to four weeks (see opposite) without making other changes. Keep a food diary and then reintroduce them (see page 27). But don't avoid them unless you have reason to believe they are at fault. They are an excellent source of nutrients, fibre and are staple foods that have been eaten around the world for millennia.

Phase 1 – Removal and Repair

This phase is to give your gut lining a chance to recover, and you should keep to it for about four weeks. The recipes – marked as '**good for Phase 1**' – are specially created for gentle repair and nourishment of the gut. They involve foods which are either low in dairy or dairy-free, low in gluten or gluten-free; and also low in the types of vegetables and pulses that are particularly high in fibre and are not digested well by some people (they end up becoming fermented further down the bowel, causing wind, pain and bloating). This phase does not contain significant amounts of fermented foods either.

If you are looking to test or confirm specific food intolerances, we would recommend you remove no more than one or two foods at a time, and ideally that you do not remove whole food groups. Common culprits implicated in gut problems include gluten, dairy, eggs, soya and coffee. You can, if necessary, repeat the process at a later date with other suspected foods.

Aim to significantly reduce or ideally avoid:

• Gluten and refined grains
• Dairy products, particularly milk
• Pulses, as the lectin in these can cause bloating (though these can be reintroduced after two weeks in vegetarians to maintain protein intake)
• Very fibrous vegetables containing lots of insoluble fibre, such as kale stalks or stringy beans
• Alcohol and puddings (sorry)

Do include plenty of:

• Non-fibrous, plant-based foods, enough to fill over half your plate, aiming for at least seven portions of veg and fruit a day, mainly made up of veg – and make them colourful too
• Good-quality proteins, to aid repair of the gut lining – aim for at least 45-60g a day
• Bitter leaf and citrus salads to boost digestion before a meal
• Non-dairy fats, such as olive oil and coconut oil, as well as avocados, nuts and seeds

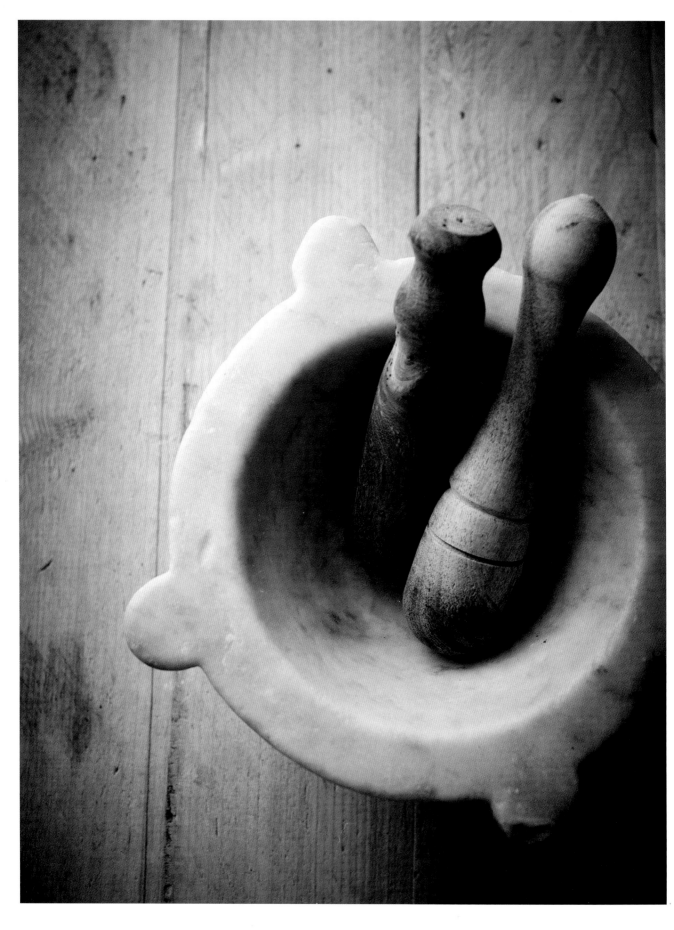

Phase 2 – Reintroduction and Recovery

In this phase, you reintroduce variety, more fibre, as well as pre- and probiotics. When you move on to Phase 2, you can choose any recipe in the book.

Increasing prebiotic foods

Prebiotics feed the good microbes (the fertiliser). The following foods are rich in prebiotics so we've included them in our recipes:

- Jerusalem artichokes, onions, leeks, garlic, fennel, asparagus, apples, pak choi
- Pulses such as lentils, peas and beans

Increasing probiotics

These are the foods that help top up the good microbes (the seeds). Start with small portions at first so your gut gets used to them:

- Fermented vegetables such as sauerkraut (page 185)
- Live yoghurts
- Kefir milk (page 190)
- Cheeses
- Kombucha to drink (page 180)

Reintroducing excluded foods

Try one food at a time, over three days. Eat a normal portion of the suspected food and if symptoms return over the next few days, withdraw that food. Allow a few days' recovery before reintroducing another food. Use the Food and Symptoms Diary to monitor your response. In the case of dairy products, you should try full-fat live yoghurt first, as this is usually best tolerated, then cheese and butter and milk last of all. If you have excluded all gluten, start with grains that contain relatively little gluten, such as rye or spelt. Sourdough breads (page 198) are easier to digest as the fermentation process breaks down much of the gluten. Then you can move on to a small amount of wheat, again over a few days.

Clever Guts Stores

Before considering which exciting new ingredients to add to your stores, we would recommend you do a quick clear-out, removing sugary processed and starchy temptations from your kitchen first – particularly if they are lurking enticingly at the front of your cupboards or on the counter tops. We don't by any means suggest that you buy all of the items listed below – this is meant to be an inspirational checklist. Buy according to the recipes that appeal to you in general, and remember the Clever Guts mantra: the greater variety of food you eat, the happier and healthier your microbiome will be. To make it easier we have shown the most commonly used ingredients in **bold**.

SPICES:

Black peppercorns
Cardamom pods
Cayenne pepper
Chilli flakes
Cinnamon, ground
Coriander, ground
**Cumin, seeds
  and ground**
Curry powder
Ginger, ground
Maldon sea salt
Mixed spice
Mustard seeds
Nutmeg
Paprika
Turmeric, ground
Vanilla essence

HERBS:
(Fresh where possible)

Bay leaves
Chives
Dill
Oregano
Parsley
Tarragon
Thyme

FLOURS AND BAKING:

Buckwheat flour
Baking powder
Bicarbonate of soda
Gram flour
Ground almonds
Rye flour
Spelt flour
Wholemeal flour
Xanthum gum

GRAINS, BEANS, PASTA AND PULSES:

Borlotti beans, canned
Black beans, canned
Brown rice
Bulgar wheat
Butterbeans, canned
Cannellini beans, canned
Chickpeas, canned
Green lentils, canned
Green-pea pasta shapes
Kidney beans, canned
Puy lentils, cooked,
  vacuum-packed
Red lentils, dried
Red rice
Rolled oats
Quinoa
Soba noodles

OILS AND VINEGARS:

Balsamic vinegar
Coconut oil
Extra-virgin olive oil
Light olive oil
Live apple cider vinegar
Mirin
Olive oil
Rapeseed oil
Rice wine vinegar
Sesame oil

FLAVOURINGS, SAUCES, SWEETENERS AND PASTES:

Basil pesto
Cacao powder
Creamed horseradish
Dark chocolate (70%)
Date syrup or 'nectar'
Desiccated coconut
Fresh root ginger
Garlic, fresh
Harissa paste
Honey
Maple syrup
Marigold stock powder
Marmite
Miso paste
Mustard, Dijon and wholegrain
Nori seaweed
Organic tea (for kombucha)
Tahini
Tamari
Tabasco
Thai fish sauce
Tomato purée
Worcestershire sauce

CANNED OR BOTTLED FOODS:

Anchovies
Artichoke hearts
Capers
Coconut cream
Coconut milk
Crab
Jalapeño peppers
Nut butters (cashew, almond)
Non-dairy milks (soy, almond)
Olives
Puréed pumpkin
Roasted red peppers
Sardines
Single soya 'cream'
Tomatoes
Tuna

NUTS AND SEEDS:

Almonds, flaked and blanched
Brazil nuts
Cashew nuts
Chia seeds
Hazelnuts
Linseeds (or flaxseed), ground
Pecan nuts
Pine nuts
Pistachio nuts
Pumpkin seeds
Sesame seeds
Sunflower seeds
Walnuts

DRIED FRUIT:

Apricots
Cranberries
Dates
Raisins
Sultanas

IN THE FRIDGE:

Raspberries, blueberries, strawberries
Butter
Buttermilk
Cheese (Parmesan, strong Cheddar, feta, halloumi)
Cream cheese
Crème fraîche
Free-range eggs
Full-fat live Greek-style yoghurt
Kefir
Lemons
Limes
Vegan Parmesan

IN THE FREEZER:

Edamame beans
Chicken breasts
Fish (salmon, cod etc)
Frozen berries
Petits pois
Prawns
Spinach

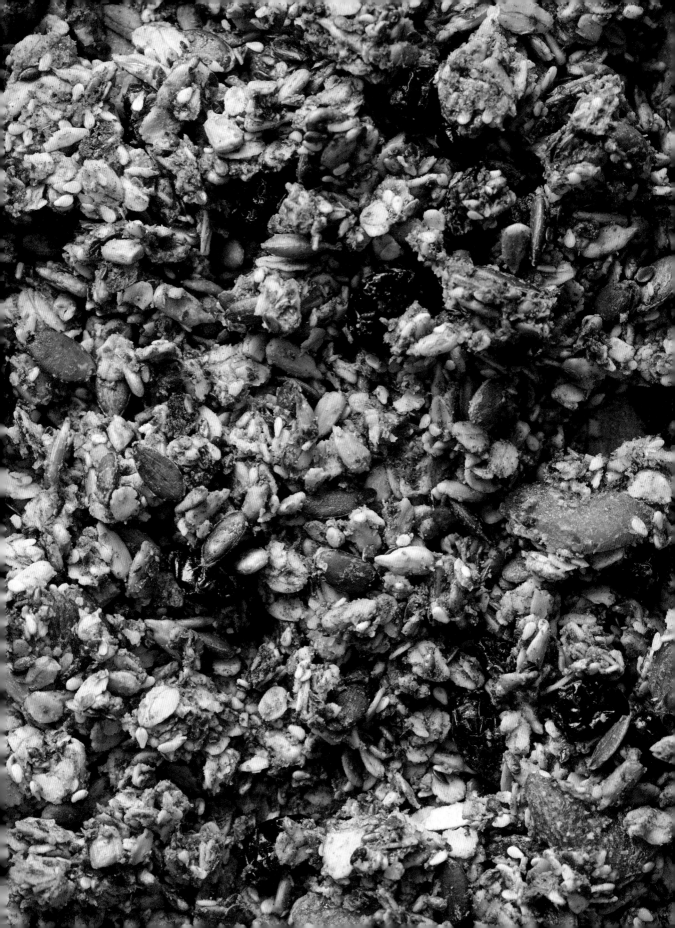

BREAKFAST

A good breakfast, eaten
mindfully, while seated,
is the best way to start
the day.

Yoghurt

Full-fat live yoghurt ticks all the Mediterranean-style healthy-eating boxes. The natural fats in it have little impact on cardiovascular disease – they may even have a beneficial effect; and its live micro-organisms feed the good bacteria in your gut. If you make your own yoghurt, then even better – you know it's going to be full of lovely live cultures. We recommend Greek-style yoghurt as the straining process increases the protein and nutrient content. But there are good non-dairy equivalents available, too.

Yoghurt with Granola and Diced Pear

We particularly enjoy this combination, which also makes an easy pudding shared between two.

Serves 1

1 small conference pear, skin on, cored and diced
100g full-fat live Greek-style yoghurt (or non-dairy equivalent)
2 tbsp Healthy Homemade Granola (page 34)

• DAIRY-FREE OPTION
• GLUTEN-FREE
• GOOD FOR PHASE 1

1. Place the diced pear in a jar or bowl.

2. Add the yoghurt and sprinkle the granola on top. **Easy.**

Tip: those of you on Phase 2 can try substituting the yoghurt for kefir, which has a delicious tartness and delivers even more good probiotics to your microbiome. To make your own kefir, see page 190. Add a drizzle of maple syrup if you find the kefir too sour, or add some diced strawberries.

440 CALORIES

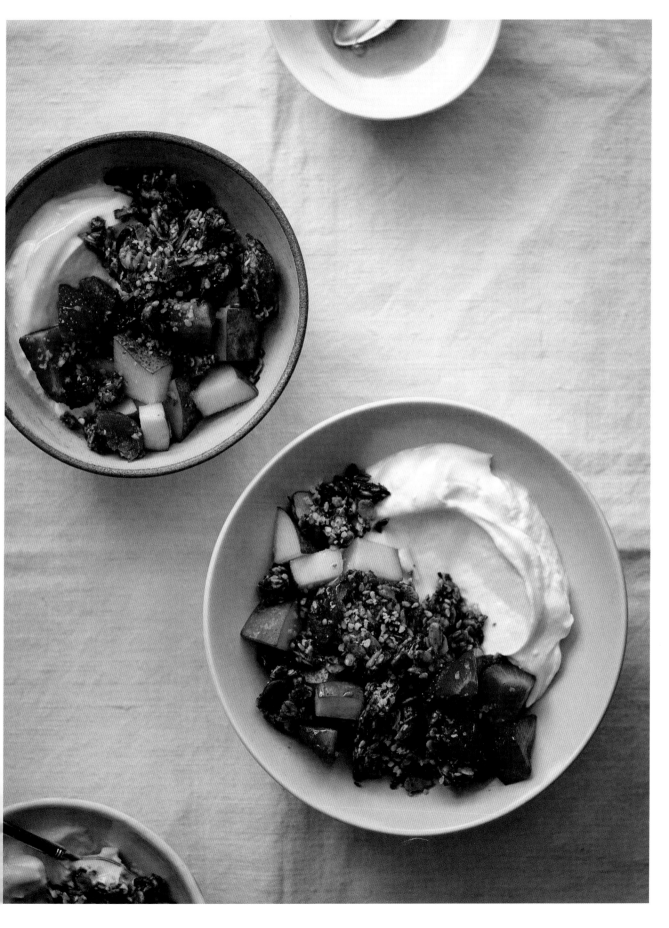

Healthy Homemade Granola

This crunchy granola is full of toasted nutty flavours. If you make it yourself you know it's gluten-free and that it's also likely to be much lower in sugar than most supermarket versions. Seeds, nuts and unprocessed oats are absorbed slowly in the gut as they are made of complex carbohydrates containing lots of fibre. And your microbiome will thrive on the fibre, too.

Makes 12 servings

100g coconut oil
   (approximately 2 heaped
   tbsp when cold/solid),
   melted
100g soft dates (about 15
   large dates), finely
   chopped
1 level tsp table salt
2 tsp vanilla essence
1 egg white, to bind
200g jumbo gluten-free
   oats (or rolled oats)
200g mixed seeds, such
   as sunflower, sesame and
   pumpkin, and nuts, such
   as almonds, cashews
   or pistachios
80g ground flaxseeds
100g dried fruit, such
   as cranberries, raisins
   or diced apricots

•DAIRY-FREE

•GLUTEN-FREE

•GOOD FOR PHASE 1

1. Preheat the oven to 120°C/100°C fan/gas mark ½. Blitz the dates, coconut oil, salt, vanilla essence and egg white in a food processor or with a hand blender to form a rough paste.

2. Put the oats, seeds, nuts, ground flaxseeds and dried fruit in a medium-sized bowl and pour in the date mixture, working it evenly into the oats with a wooden spoon.

3. Scatter the mixture in the bottom of a shallow medium-sized baking tray lined with greaseproof paper and bake it for 25-30 minutes. Then turn the oven off and leave it to crisp up for an hour or two, or even overnight, before breaking it up into small clusters. It can be stored in an airtight jar for up to a month, or in the freezer for several months.

Tip: 1-2 tbsp water can be used instead of the egg white.

340 CALORIES

Yoghurt with Chia Jam and Toasted Pistachios

Abandon those low-fat sugary yoghurts for the real thing – thick and creamy full-fat yoghurt is back on the menu as a staple in a healthy diet. The chia jam and toasted nuts here will give you all the sweetness you need.

Serves 1

1 tbsp chia jam (page 208)

100g full-fat live Greek-
    style yoghurt (or non-
    dairy equivalent)

Handful of berries, such
    as raspberries,
    strawberries or
    blueberries

1 tbsp toasted nuts, such
    as pistachios or almonds

• DAIRY-FREE OPTION
• GLUTEN-FREE
• GOOD FOR PHASE 1

1. Spoon the chia jam into a glass or small jar.

2. Dollop the yoghurt on top, and then sprinkle with the berries and toasted nuts.

230 CALORIES

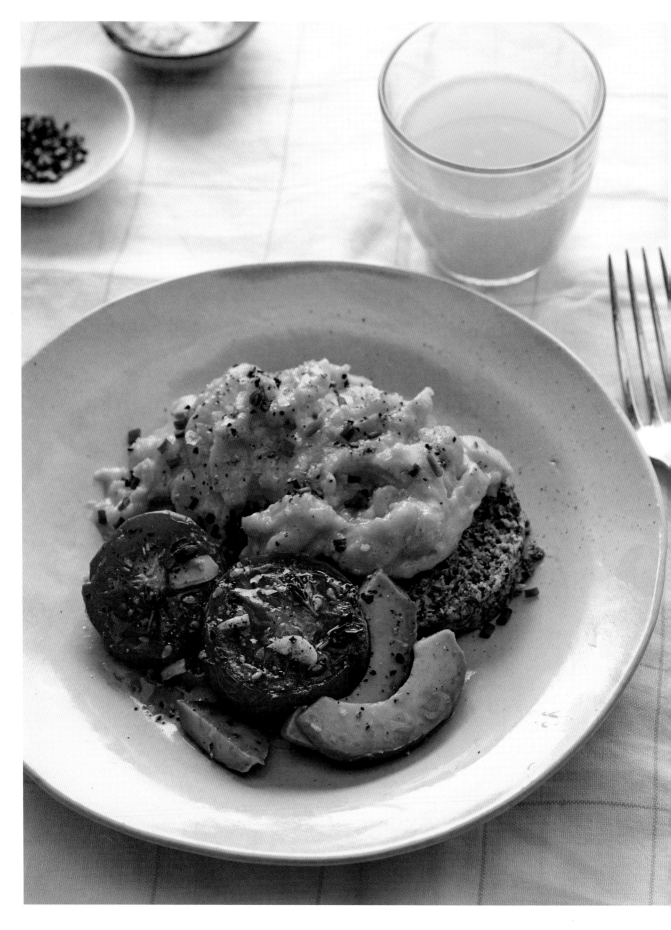

Eggs

Michael and I love eggs. Fears that they raise cholesterol are unfounded. Embrace them. Enjoy them. See how good you feel going to work on an egg.

Simple Creamy Scrambled Eggs

Serves 1
2 eggs
Small knob of butter or
    drizzle of oil

• DAIRY-FREE
• GLUTEN-FREE
• GOOD FOR PHASE 1

1. Whisk the eggs with a fork in a cup or small bowl.

2. In a small non-stick saucepan, melt the butter over a low heat, without allowing it to brown. Pour in the eggs and stir gently with a wooden spoon for 1-2 minutes.

3. Remove the eggs from the heat when they start to thicken but are still a bit runny in places. Don't overcook them or they will be rubbery. Transfer them immediately to the plate.

4. Scatter some Maldon sea salt and freshly ground pepper or a pinch of chilli flakes on top. You can jazz them up with a few fresh herbs, such as chopped chives, too.

190 CALORIES

With smoked salmon: top with 50g smoked salmon, a squeeze of lemon and ground black pepper to taste (add 90 cals).

With leafy veg and Parmesan: add a handful of cooked leftover greens and 20g grated Parmesan (or vegan Parmesan) as you scramble the eggs (add 100 cals).

With chestnut mushrooms: fry the mushrooms in oil or butter for 4-5 minutes. Season, scatter with chopped parsley, and serve them alongside the scrambled eggs (add 60 cals, plus another 60 cals if you use ½ tbsp oil for frying).

On a slice of toast: try your scrambled eggs on a slice of toasted Mug Bread (page 94; see pic, *left*) or Sourdough (page 198) with butter (add 300 cals).

Turmeric Spiced Omelette with Seaweed

Give your omelette an extra kick with this spiced coconut mixture, which contains two fabulously gut-friendly ingredients, turmeric and seaweed.

Serves 2

Small knob of butter
  or drizzle of oil
4 medium mushrooms,
  finely chopped
4 eggs
1 tbsp Dry Coconut Sambal
  (page 120)
Freshly ground black
  pepper

• DAIRY-FREE OPTION
• GLUTEN-FREE
• GOOD FOR PHASE 1

1. Heat the butter or oil in a small frying pan and sauté the mushrooms for around 5 minutes or until they are soft.

2. Beat the eggs in a bowl and pour them into the pan. Lower the heat, scatter the coconut sambal on top and cook until the bottom of the omelette is starting to firm up but the top is still moist. Fold the omelette over, cut it in half and serve it immediately.

Tip: ground black pepper massively enhances the benefit of turmeric.

270 CALORIES

Mushroom Omelette with Red Sauerkraut

Sauerkraut works well added to an omelette, providing a salty, tangy crunch, and lots of good bugs for your microbiome.

Serves 1

Small knob of butter
  or drizzle of oil
2 medium chestnut
  mushrooms, finely diced
2 eggs
1 tbsp Red Cabbage
  Sauerkraut (page 185)

• DAIRY-FREE
• GLUTEN-FREE

1. Heat the butter or oil in a small frying pan and sauté the mushrooms for around 5 minutes or until they are soft.

2. Beat the eggs in a bowl and pour them into the pan. Lower the heat and cook until the bottom of the omelette is starting to firm up but the top is still moist. Fold the omelette over and transfer it to a plate.

3. Spread the sauerkraut on top, and serve with freshly ground black pepper.

Tip: for Phase 1 skip the sauerkraut.

220 CALORIES

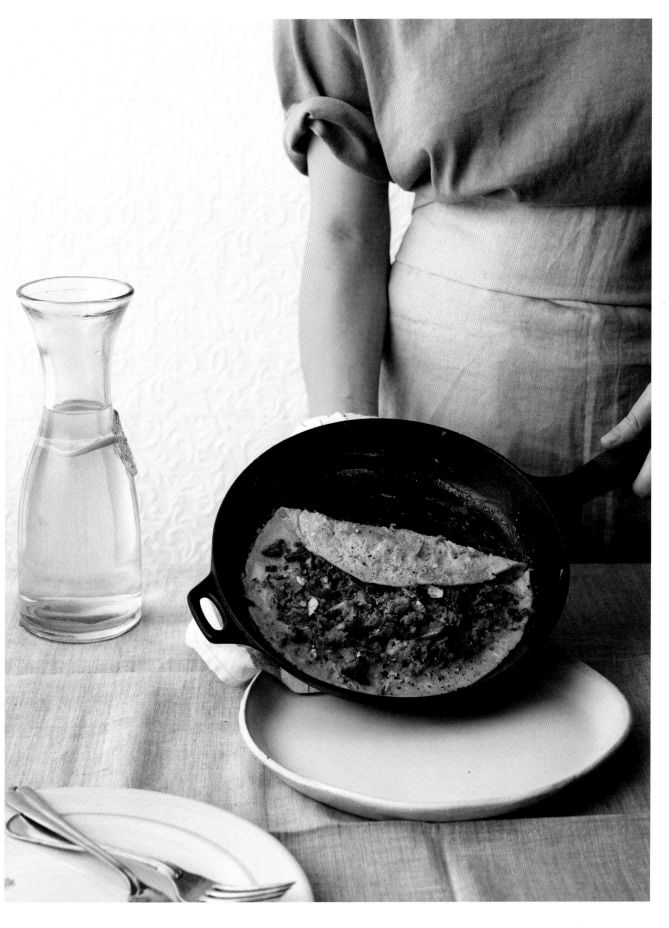

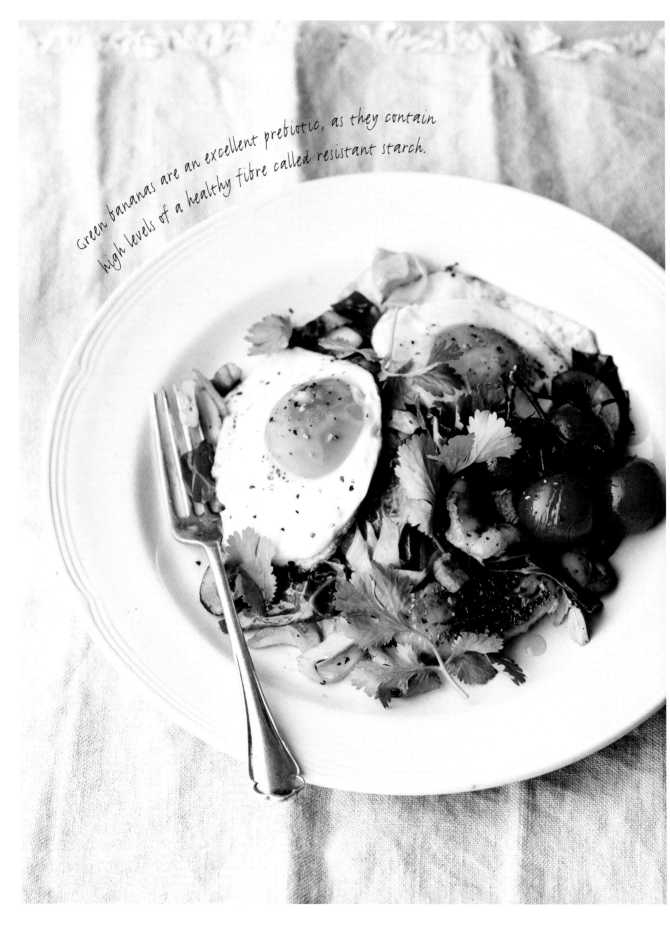

Green bananas are an excellent prebiotic, as they contain high levels of a healthy fibre called resistant starch.

Breakfast Fry-Up with Green Bananas

Our kids have turned breakfast fry-ups into a well-honed art form, cooked with more enthusiasm than almost any other meal. Try this gut-friendly version, made with green bananas which are made up of an astonishing 70-80% resistant starch. (Sadly this drops to only 1% in ripe bananas as the starch gets converted into simple sugars – sucrose, glucose and fructose.) I got to love fried green bananas after eating them for breakfast every day while working on a medical project in the Amazon jungle.

Serves 2

60g pancetta cubes
  or diced bacon
2-3 tbsp olive oil
120g mushrooms, sliced
1 large green banana,
  halved lengthways
2 eggs
150g small plum tomatoes,
  halved
150g cooked cabbage or
  kale, chopped and tough
  stalks removed (leftover
  greens are ideal)
½ tsp ground nutmeg

• DAIRY-FREE
• GLUTEN-FREE
• GOOD FOR PHASE 1

1. Place the pancetta in a small frying pan over a medium heat and fry it for around 5 minutes, or until it is brown and crispy, then set it aside.

2. Pour the olive oil into another, larger frying pan and fry the mushrooms and banana over a medium heat. Season with salt and pepper. Clear a space in the middle of the pan, add a little more oil if necessary and crack in the eggs.

3. Season the greens and add them to the pan with the tomatoes and nutmeg, then scatter the pancetta on top. Cook everything for a couple more minutes – the egg yolk should still be a bit runny. Serve the fry-up on warm plates.

Tip: keep the green banana in the fridge so it does not ripen and convert to sugars.

440 CALORIES

Porridge

Bin those processed breakfast cereals, most of which are stuffed with hidden sugars. That also includes instant porridge sachets, which contain little of the complex carbohydrate or fibre needed by your microbiome. Our porridge recipes use whole oats, which are only minimally processed and still contain the nutritious inner kernel of the oats, along with plenty of fibre and nutrients to keep you going well into the day.

Coconut Porridge with Pecans and Pear

A creamy, nutty porridge laced with sweet juicy pear.

Serves 2

50g rolled oats (or gluten-
  free oats)
200ml coconut milk
½ tsp ground cinnamon
¼ tsp ground nutmeg
Pinch of salt
20g pecan nuts, roughly
  chopped
½ pear, cored and diced

•DAIRY-FREE
•GLUTEN-FREE OPTION
•GOOD FOR PHASE 1

1. Place the oats, coconut milk, spices, salt and pecans in a small pan and bring it to a simmer. Cook gently for 10-12 minutes, stirring frequently, until the mixture is thick and creamy.

2. Pour it into a bowl, scatter the diced pear on top and dig in. A teaspoonful of honey won't harm, but it's just as good without...

370 CALORIES

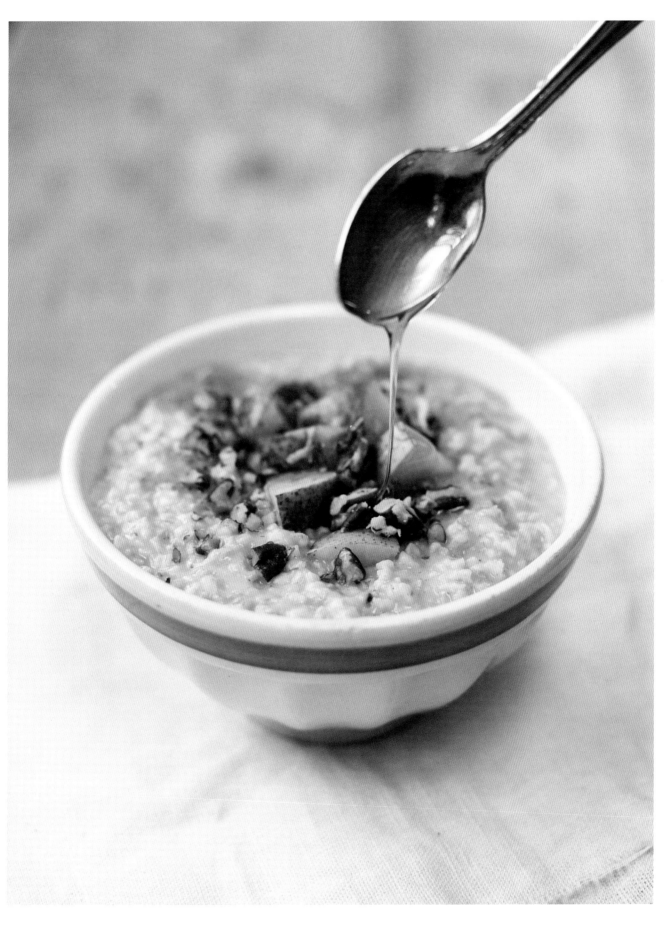

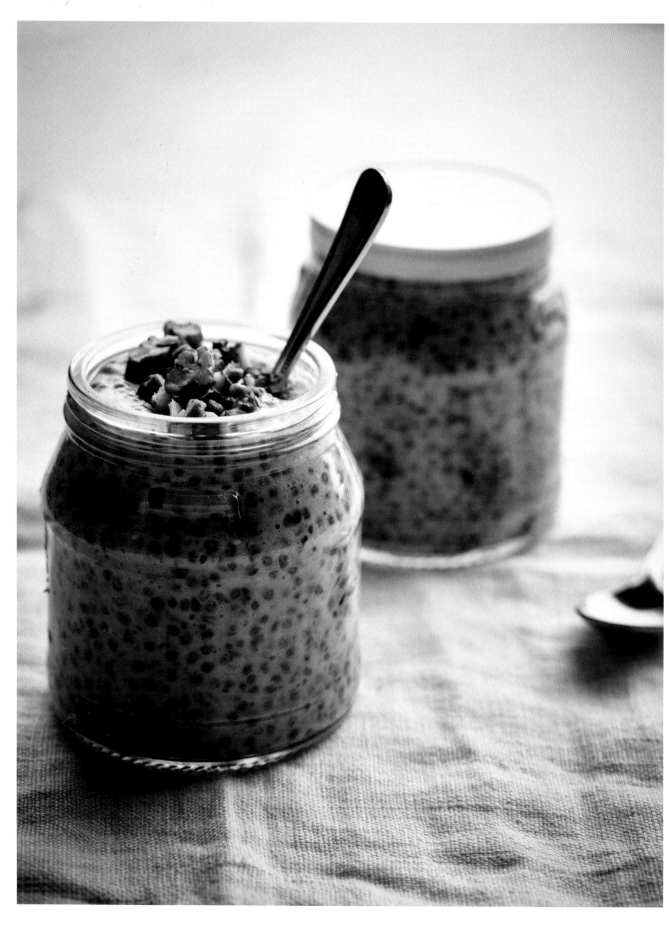

Blueberry Chia Pots

Serves 2

400ml can coconut milk
3 tbsp chia seeds
1 tsp vanilla essence
1 tsp ground nutmeg
Juice of 1 large lemon
225g blueberries
3 tbsp pecan nuts,
   roughly chopped

•DAIRY-FREE
•GLUTEN-FREE
•GOOD FOR PHASE 1

1. With a food processor or hand blender, blitz the coconut milk, chia, vanilla and nutmeg for about 1 minute or until you have a smooth creamy mixture. Add the lemon juice and blueberries and pulse briefly – you want to retain some texture.

2. Spoon the mixture into pots or bowls and leave it to thicken in the fridge overnight or for at least 30 minutes.

3. When you are ready to eat it, scatter the pecans on top.

Tip: this also makes a great pudding – divide it into 4 portions and halve the calorie count.

590 CALORIES

Bircher Muesli with Kefir

Serves 4

400g rolled oats
50g cashew nuts
25g sesame seeds
25g pumpkin seeds
25g desiccated coconut
25g dried cranberries
400ml almond milk
   (or dairy milk if using)
150ml kefir
   (or non-dairy equivalent)
150g berries, such as
   blueberries or raspberries

•DAIRY-FREE OPTION
•GOOD FOR PHASE 1

1. Put the oats in a bowl or glass jar with the cashew nuts, sesame and pumpkin seeds, desiccated coconut and cranberries. Stir in the milk and store it in the fridge, covered, overnight. (Soaking muesli helps to break down the cell walls in the seeds, nuts and fruits, making them easier to digest.)

2. Before serving, stir in the kefir and scatter the berries on top.

Tip: store it in the fridge or freeze extra portions for another day.

660 CALORIES

Oily Fish

Oily fish works wonders in your gut and is one of the best possible sources of omega 3 – something we need to eat more of to create a healthy balance with the more readily available omega 6 oils. Oily fish helps to keep down blood sugars, too.

Avocado and Smoked Salmon

Simple, high in protein and omega 3 oils, this is a great breakfast that will keep you full for the rest of the morning.

Serves 2
1 avocado, finely sliced
160g smoked salmon
Juice of ½ lemon

• DAIRY-FREE
• GLUTEN-FREE
• GOOD FOR PHASE 1

1. Divide the avocado between two plates, fanning the slices out.

2. Place the smoked salmon on top with a generous squeeze of lemon juice and a grinding of black pepper. Serve immediately.

280 CALORIES

Speedy Kippers with Blistered Tomatoes

One of the healthiest and best-value breakfasts available.

Serves 2
1 pack boil-in-the-bag kippers
8 cherry tomatoes, halved

• DAIRY-FREE
• GLUTEN-FREE
• GOOD FOR PHASE 1

1. Microwave or boil the kippers according to the pack instructions.

2. Put the tomatoes in a non-stick frying pan on a high heat, cut side up for about 3 minutes until the skins are blistered. Serve immediately.

270 CALORIES

Smoked Mackerel and Kale Kedgeree

So quick to make and so tasty, with turmeric for added flavour and a healthy anti-inflammatory boost.

Serves 4

125g brown basmati rice
2 tbsp olive oil
1 onion, diced
½ red pepper, deseeded
   and diced
1 tsp curry powder
½ tsp turmeric
165g cauliflower, broken
   into florets
2 handfuls of kale, shredded
3 smoked mackerel fillets,
   skinned and broken
   into chunks
4 eggs, hardboiled, halved

•DAIRY-FREE
•GLUTEN-FREE
•GOOD FOR PHASE 1

1. Cook the rice according to the pack instructions, ideally the night before. Leave it to chill in the fridge.

2. Meanwhile, heat the oil in a large frying pan and sauté the onion and pepper for 4-5 minutes. Stir in the spices and cook for another minute, before adding the cauliflower and rice.

3. Cook for a further 2-3 minutes, stirring occasionally, then add the kale and smoked mackerel and cook for a further 4-5 minutes, until the kale has wilted and the mackerel is heated through.

4. Gently stir the eggs into the kedgeree and season to taste before serving.

540 CALORIES

Clever Smoothies

Nutrient-rich shakes make a great one-stop meal for those who don't feel like eating first thing in the morning or don't have time for breakfast. If you blitz them less, they retain more texture, ensuring that you still get plenty of healthy fibre for those bugs to get their teeth into. The natural fats we have included will help you feel satiated without spiking your blood sugars. They will also improve the absorption of fat-soluble vitamins.

Clever Guts Green Smoothie

A satisfying start to the day, full of green goodness.

Serves 1

4 celery stalks, chopped
Small handful of kale, chopped, tough stalks removed
Large handful of spinach
2 pak choi, tops only
½ avocado, sliced
80g blueberries
2 tbsp full-fat live Greek-style yoghurt (or non-dairy equivalent)
1 tbsp olive oil
Handful of ice cubes

• DAIRY-FREE OPTION
• GLUTEN-FREE
• GOOD FOR PHASE 1

1. Place all the ingredients in a blender with 200ml water and blitz for 10-20 seconds. The mixture should retain a little texture.

2. Pour it into a jug and store it in the fridge. It will keep for up to 24 hours.

Note: if you have IBS you might wish to reduce the amount of celery.

450 CALORIES

These drinks are ideal to keep you going on a fast day –
one serving will provide about half of your daily calorie count,
the rest of which you can make up with a meal.

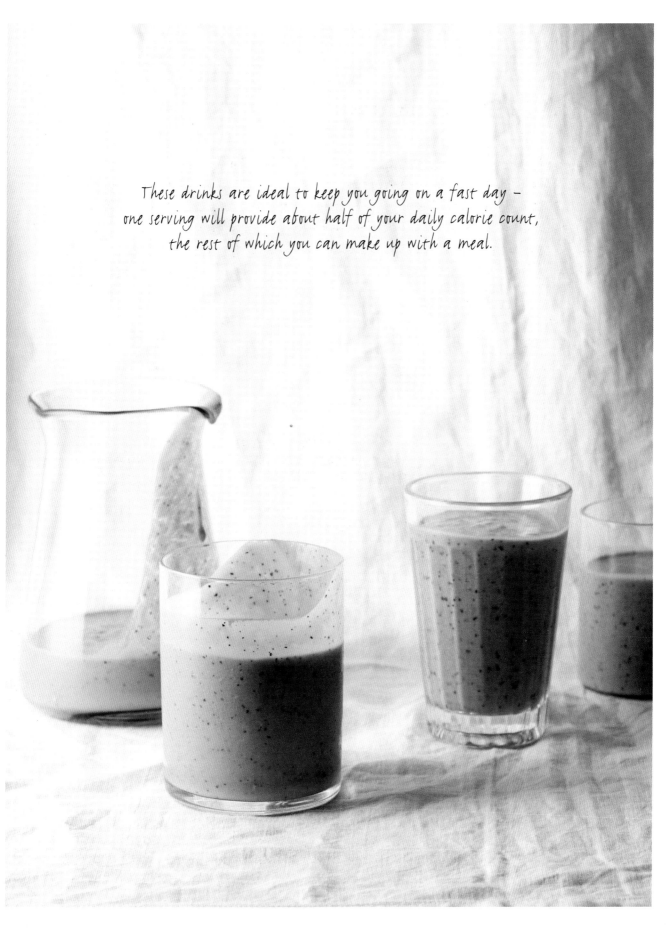

Dr Tim's Healthy Gut Smoothie

A thick, fruity smoothie shared by our great friend Tim in Australia, who slimmed back down to the figure he had at medical school by drinking these as part of his 5:2 fast day regimen.

Serves 1

½ avocado, sliced

1 apple, cored and chopped

2 pak choi, green leaves only

1 tbsp olive oil

2 tbsp full-fat live Greek-style yogurt (or non-dairy equivalent)

3 tbsp dairy or non-dairy milk, such as almond or soya

Large handful of spinach leaves

75g frozen strawberries or blueberries

Handful of ice cubes

•DAIRY-FREE OPTION

•GLUTEN-FREE

•GOOD FOR PHASE 1

1. Place all the ingredients in a blender and blitz for 10-20 seconds. The mixture should retain a little texture.

2. Pour it into a jug and store it in the fridge. It will keep for up to 24 hours.

520 CALORIES

Creamy Pineapple Smoothie

Pineapple is one of the surprise ingredients of the Clever Guts Diet. Not only is it rich in fibre, it also contains an enzyme called bromelain which helps digestion, particularly of protein, and is thought to have anti-inflammatory properties.

Serves 2

325g fresh pineapple, skin
   removed, chopped
50g cashew nuts
50g sunflower seeds
200ml kefir or buttermilk
   (or non-dairy equivalent)
125ml almond milk
Pinch of ground cinnamon

• DAIRY-FREE OPTION
• GLUTEN-FREE
• GOOD FOR PHASE 1

Place all the ingredients in a blender and blitz until you have a fairly smooth mixture. Serve it immediately.

Tip: if your blender does not break down nuts or seeds easily, try soaking them in the milk for an hour first.

460 CALORIES

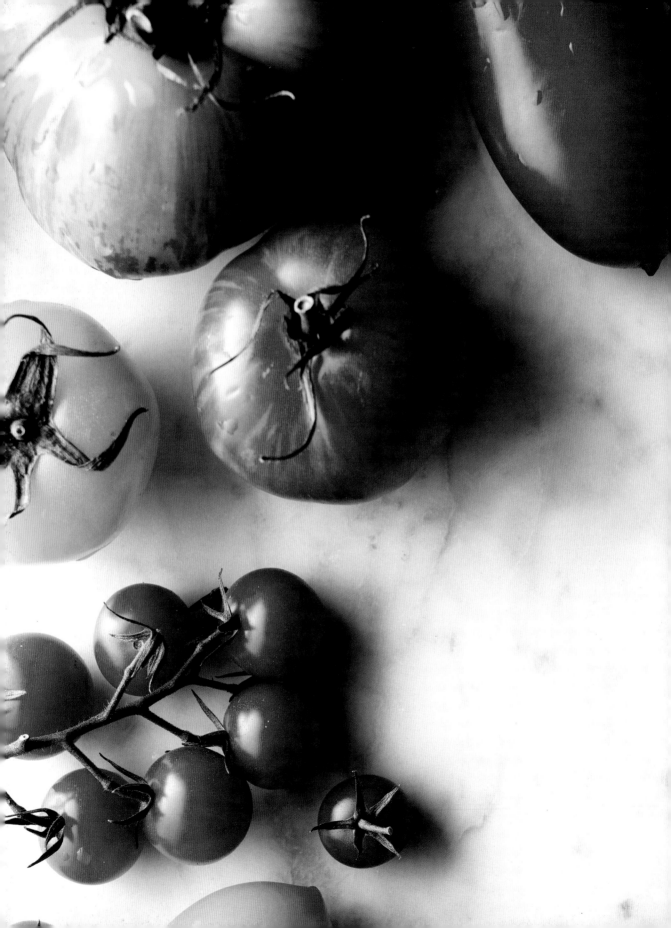

LIGHT MEALS, SOUPS AND SALADS

Enzyme-stimulating salads, healing broths, gut-friendly snacks and a range of simple, tasty dishes to expand your daily repertoire and nurture your good bacteria...

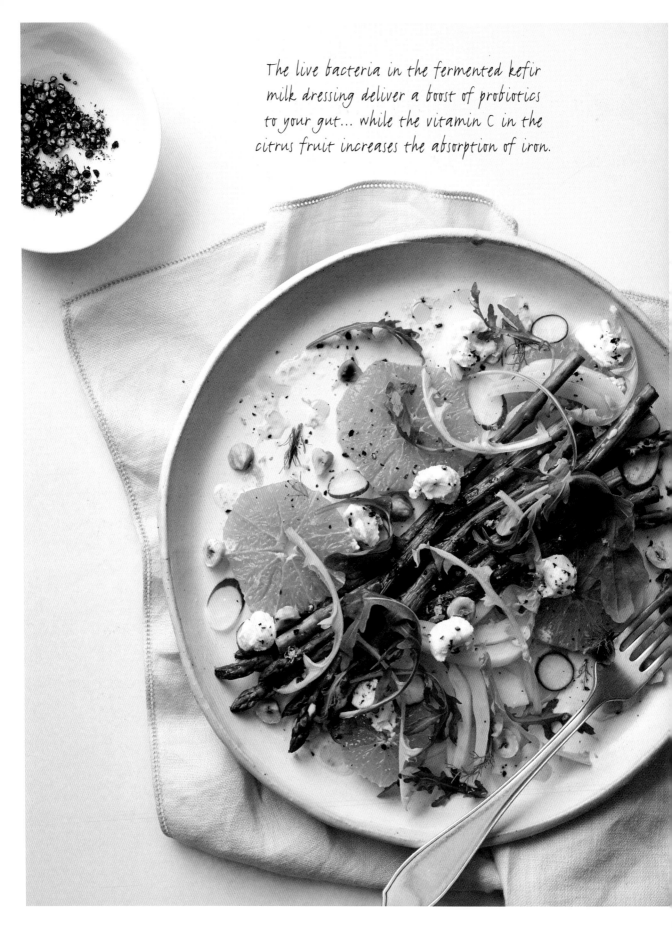

The live bacteria in the fermented kefir milk dressing deliver a boost of probiotics to your gut... while the vitamin C in the citrus fruit increases the absorption of iron.

Enzyme-stimulating Salads

Eating bitter leaves, such as rocket, watercress or spinach, or sharp citrus fruits before or with your main meal helps get the digestive process going.

Citrus, Fennel and Asparagus Salad

Serves 2
8 large asparagus spears
1 large orange, sliced
1 fennel bulb, halved
   and thinly sliced
2 handfuls of bitter leaves
4 tbsp Lemon Buttermilk
   Dressing (page 118)

•GLUTEN-FREE
•GOOD FOR PHASE 1

1. Sear the asparagus on a very hot griddle for 4-5 minutes, turning it frequently, then transfer it to a plate and slice it in half lengthways.

2. Place all the other ingredients in a salad bowl and toss them together with the dressing.

Tip: to make this salad more substantial you can add 40g crumbled goat's cheese and 50g toasted hazelnuts (add 250 cals per portion).

100 CALORIES

Blood Orange Salad with Toasted Coriander

Serves 2
1 blood orange
Small bunch of watercress
½ red onion, finely sliced
1 tsp coriander seeds
4 tbsp olive oil
Juice of ½ lemon

•DAIRY-FREE
•GLUTEN-FREE
•GOOD FOR PHASE 1

1. Break the orange into segments, and place them with the watercress and red onion in a salad bowl.

2. Toast and lightly crush the coriander seeds, and then make a dressing by whisking them together with the olive oil and lemon juice. Pour it over the salad and toss well before serving.

280 CALORIES

Bitter Leaves and Toasted Pine Nut Salad

One of our top ten Clever Guts ingredients, apple cider vinegar has been shown to reduce blood sugars and even encourage weight loss in some individuals. It contains a host of live microbiome-enhancing micro-organisms – if left in the cupboard it may grow wispy strands and form a 'mother' made up of proteins, enzymes, bacteria and yeasts, which only enhance the benefits.

Serves 2

3 tbsp olive oil

1 tbsp live apple cider vinegar

2 generous handfuls
of rocket, watercress,
dandelion or baby
spinach, or a mixture of
leaves

1 tbsp Parmesan shavings
(or vegan Parmesan)

2 tbsp pine nuts, toasted

• DAIRY-FREE OPTION

• GLUTEN-FREE

• GOOD FOR PHASE 1

1. To make the dressing, whisk together the olive oil and cider vinegar and season with Maldon sea salt and black pepper.

2. Place the salad leaves in a bowl, and toss them in the dressing.

3. Sprinkle the Parmesan shavings and toasted pine nuts on top before serving.

Tip: for a more filling salad add 50g fresh marinated anchovies, available from most supermarkets. They will not only add flavour, but also tick the oily fish box (add about 35 cals).

260 CALORIES

Cider Vinegar Tipple

If you don't have time for a salad, you can simply drink a diluted 'gin-and-tonic' sized portion of this before a meal to stimulate digestion.

Serves 1

½-1 tbsp live apple cider
vinegar

150-200ml water

• DAIRY-FREE

• GLUTEN-FREE

Add the vinegar to either warm or cold water. You can make it a bit stronger than this, but don't overdo it; it is not currently recommended to have more than 2 tbsp vinegar a day.

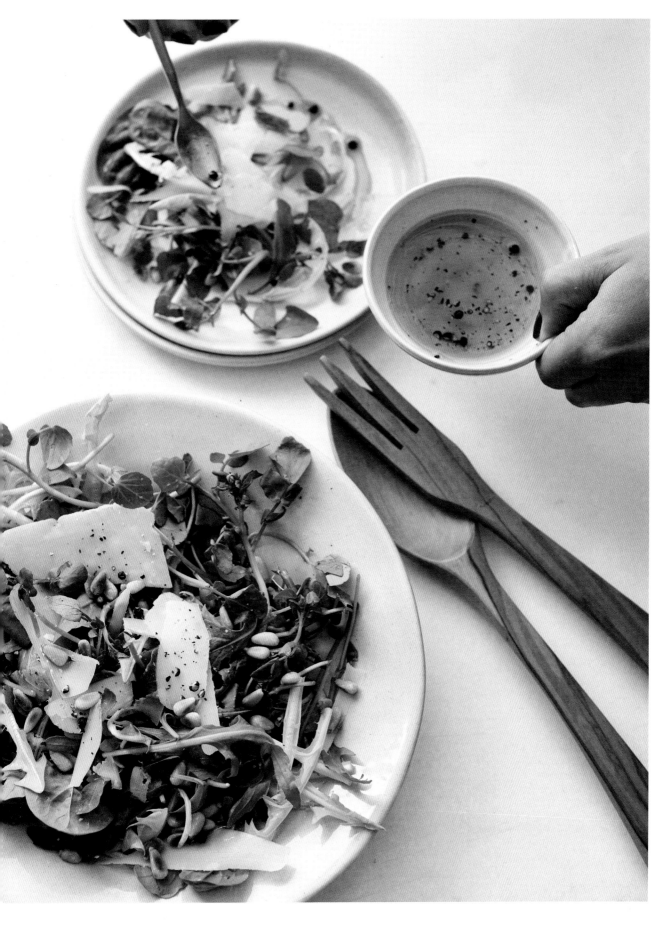

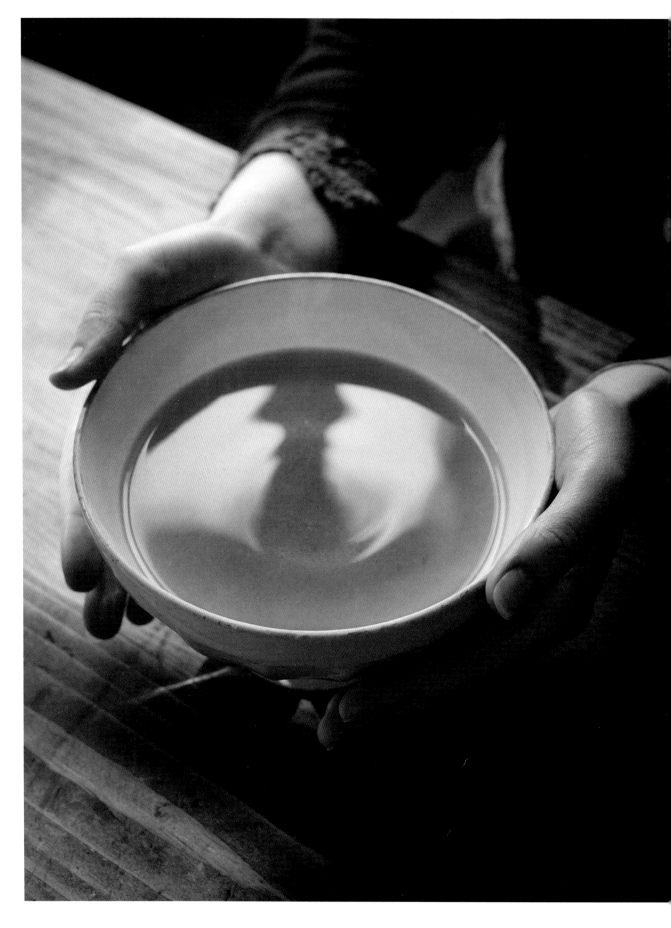

Broths and Soups

Broths, which are slow-cooked to release minerals and nutrients from bones, are wonderfully nourishing for the gut. Soup, meanwhile, has the magical ability to reduce blood sugar spikes that would be caused by eating its individual ingredients separately, so offering maximum nutrition while keeping you full for longer. This is because the food is emulsified and therefore digested more slowly. A bowl of steaming soup enhances life.

Healing Chicken Bone Broth

A classic 'medicinal' food, used all over the world to soothe troubled guts and aid recovery after illness. A perfect way to use up leftover chicken bones.

Makes approx 2 litres, serves 8

3 tbsp olive oil
4 celery stalks, roughly chopped
2 small onions, chopped
2 leeks, trimmed
1 large garlic clove, halved
2 carrots, chopped
1kg chicken wings and/or chicken carcasses (ideally organic)
1 tbsp live apple cider vinegar (ideally organic)
2 bay leaves
1 bouquet garni
Handful of parsley stalks
6-8 black peppercorns

• DAIRY-FREE
• GLUTEN-FREE
• GOOD FOR PHASE 1

1. Heat the oil in a large pan with a lid and sauté the celery, onions and leeks for 5-7 minutes. Add the garlic, carrots, chicken, cider vinegar, bay leaves, bouquet garni and parsley.

2. Pour in 2-2.5 litres of water and bring everything to a gentle simmer, then cover the pan and cook gently for at least 3 hours, ideally for 5-6 hours, to get the most nutrients from the bones.

3. Check occasionally to ensure that it has not dried out and top up with water if needed, skimming any scum from the surface.

4. Place a sieve over a large bowl and pour the stock through it, allowing it to drip for 15 minutes. For a thicker, tastier broth you can gently press the soft vegetables through the sieve with a spoon.

5. Either use it immediately or let it cool, then ladle it into containers and keep it in the fridge for up to 5 days. It can also be frozen.

40 CALORIES

Gut-Soothing Vegetable Bouillon

This classic vegetable stock makes an excellent clear soup, and can also be used as a tasty and nutritious base for all sorts of recipes, from stews or casseroles to sauces. It can be kept in the fridge for 5 days or frozen in portions ready to use when needed.

Makes approx 1 litre, serves 4

2 tbsp olive oil

1 large onion, halved and roughly chopped

100g carrots, roughly chopped

100g leeks, trimmed and cut into 3-4cm pieces

100g celery, cut into 3-4cm pieces

Large handful of fresh parsley, including stalks

2 garlic cloves

3 bay leaves

8-10 black peppercorns

1 level tbsp Maldon sea salt

• DAIRY-FREE

• GLUTEN-FREE

• GOOD FOR PHASE 1

1. Heat the oil in a large pan and sauté the onion gently for 4-5 minutes or until it is soft. Add the remaining ingredients, along with approx 1-1.5 litres water and bring everything to the boil. Cover the pan and allow it to simmer gently for 1-1½ hours.

2. Place a sieve over a large bowl and pour the stock through it. To boost the flavour and get a thicker broth, gently press the soft vegetables through the sieve with a spoon.

3. The stock can be stored in the fridge for up to a week, or in the freezer.

20 CALORIES

Quick Seaweed Miso Soup

Ideal for a 5:2 fast day, this excellent seaweed broth was suggested by Fatrabbit, a member of the Clever Guts Forum, as a low-calorie drink that is surprisingly filling and packed with nutrients. Both Marmite and miso involve fermentation. Marmite is made from spent yeast. Miso is a traditional Japanese seasoning produced by fermenting soybeans with salt and koji, a yeast fermentation starter, and sometimes with rice, barley, or other ingredients. Neither may be suitable if you are very gluten-sensitive as they can contain small amounts of gluten; however, gluten-free equivalents are available.

Serves 1

1 tbsp dried seaweed (such as nori), chopped

1 tsp Marmite, or miso paste

• DAIRY-FREE
• GLUTEN-FREE OPTION

Place the seaweed and Marmite or miso in a mug and top up with boiling water. Leave it to stand for 1-2 minutes before drinking it.

15 CALORIES

Spicy Lentil and Tomato Soup

This comforting and fibre-rich soup is easily made using Vegetable-Rich Tomato Sauce (page 168) and Gut-Soothing Vegetable Bouillon (page 60). Lentils are added for extra protein and fibre.

Serves 2

325g Vegetable-Rich
   Tomato Sauce
50g red lentils
500ml Gut-Soothing
   Vegetable Bouillon (or
   stock of your choice)
¼ tsp chilli flakes (optional)
Small handful of fresh
   coriander, chopped

• DAIRY-FREE
• GLUTEN-FREE

1. Place the tomato sauce, lentils, vegetable bouillon and chilli flakes in a medium-sized pan and bring it to a simmer. Cook gently for 30 minutes or until the lentils are soft.

2. Scatter the chopped coriander on top just before serving.

Tip: to make this soup more filling, drizzle with 1/2 tbsp extra-virgin olive oil (add 60 cals), grate in a matchbox-sized piece of cheese (add 160 cals), scatter 1/2 tbsp toasted seeds on top (add 60 cals) or add 1 tbsp chopped fried chorizo (add 90 cals).

160 CALORIES

Green Gazpacho with Seaweed

A chilled, green, gut-friendly soup in which the seaweed adds a subtle savoury flavour along with some extra health-boosting omega 3.

Serves 2

75g watercress or baby spinach leaves

½ cucumber, roughly chopped

2 tomatoes, halved

½ green chilli, deseeded and roughly chopped

1 garlic clove, chopped

2 large nori seaweed sheets, sliced (optional)

2 spring onions, trimmed and roughly chopped

1 avocado, halved

3 tbsp extra-virgin olive oil

1 tbsp apple cider vinegar

Small handful of fresh mint and parsley leaves, roughly chopped

• DAIRY-FREE

• GLUTEN-FREE

• GOOD FOR PHASE 1

1. Place the watercress, cucumber, tomatoes, chilli, garlic, nori, spring onions and avocado in a food processor and blend until everything has broken down a little.

2. Add the olive oil and cider vinegar and pulse again. Slowly pour in 150-250ml cold water until you reach your desired consistency, and season well to taste.

3. Serve the gazpacho in bowls with a drizzle of olive oil, a few ice cubes and a sprinkling of mint and parsley.

380 CALORIES

Pink Celeriac and Beetroot Soup

Knobbly and a bit awkward to handle, celeriac needs only the minimum of peeling, as most of the nutrients are concentrated just beneath the skin. Like beetroot, it is full of the kind of complex carbohydrates loved by your gut biome. The delicate flavours of the two root vegetables combine beautifully here to make a creamy and filling soup.

Serves 4

3 tbsp olive oil

1 small onion, chopped

350g beetroot, peeled and chopped into 1½-2cm cubes

800g celeriac, peeled and chopped into 1½-2cm cubes

2cm root ginger, diced

Juice of ½ lemon

¼ -½ tsp chilli flakes

1 litre vegetable stock, or Gut-Soothing Vegetable Bouillon (page 60)

Grated cheese or toasted nuts to serve (optional)

• DAIRY-FREE

• GLUTEN-FREE

• GOOD FOR PHASE 1

1. Heat the oil in a medium-sized pan and sauté the onion for around 5 minutes or until it has softened.

2. Add the beetroot, celeriac, ginger, lemon juice and chilli flakes, then pour in the stock. Bring it to the boil and simmer, covered, for around 20 minutes, or until the vegetables are tender.

3. Purée it with a hand blender, adding more stock if you like a looser consistency. Season to taste and serve topped with a matchbox-sized piece of cheese, grated (add 160 cals), or a few toasted nuts (add 60 cals).

210 CALORIES

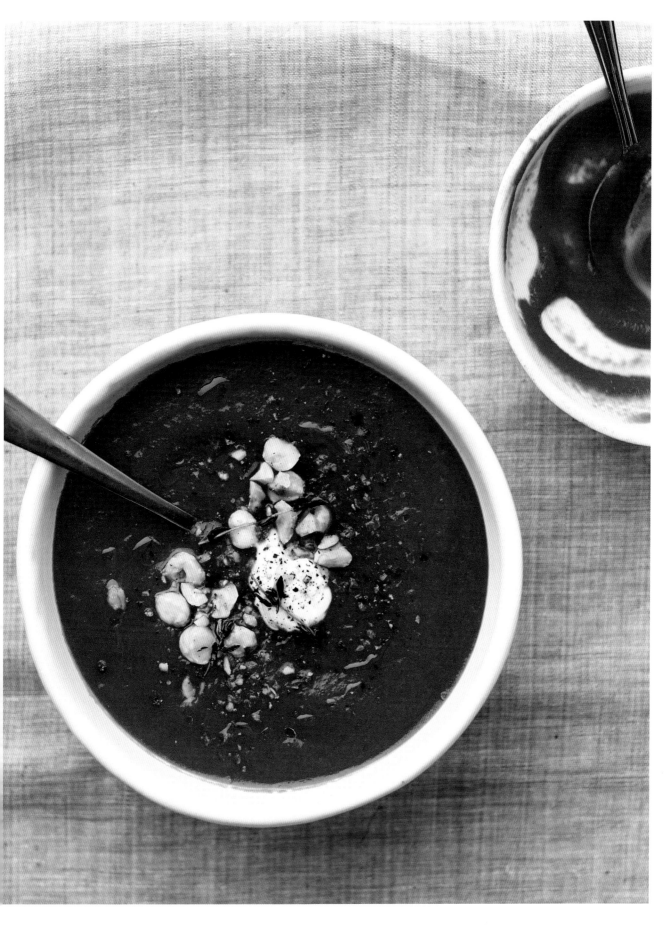

Food to Go, Dips, Spreads and Crackers

As a GP, I see many patients in whom there is a strong link between gut problems, being overweight or having type 2 diabetes and busy working lifestyles. It is not easy to find healthy snacks when on the move, and people find themselves grabbing whatever's quickest – often processed, sweet or starchy food. I hope some of these easy and practical suggestions might help you to break this cycle. Prepare them in advance to save you time in the morning. They will make you feel full for longer and your microbiome will reward you for it!

Phyto Salad

This salad will provide you with plenty of those all-important anti-inflammatory phytonutrients. While at least three-quarters of your bowl should be plant-based, you should also ensure you get the required fats and proteins. We suggest you choose something from each group below.

3-4 portions of coloured vegetables (one of which can be substituted with fruit), such as:
1 sliced carrot
½ sliced pepper (red, orange, yellow)
½ sliced courgette
5 baby tomatoes
4 steamed asparagus spears
3-4 artichoke or palm hearts
½ cup of radishes, mange touts or mushrooms
Fruit (approx ½ cup): strawberries, unpeeled pear or apple, papaya, mango, grapes, pomegranate, blueberries or raspberries

1-2 cups of greens, such as:
Spinach, mixed salad leaves, rocket, kale, broccoli, chicory, cauliflower, pak choi, sprouts, Swiss chard, cabbage

1-2 portions of protein, such as:

2 hardboiled eggs

Meat: chicken, turkey, cold meat (about 80g)

Oily fish: tuna, salmon, mackerel, sardines; or white fish, such as trout, cod, haddock (about 100g)

Dairy: hard cheese, halloumi, goat's cheese, feta (30-60g)

Plant protein: a generous handful of lentils, beans (reduce both of these if you suffer from IBS or bloating), nuts, seeds, tofu, tempeh, hummus

2-3 portions of health-boosting fats, such as:

½ small avocado

6 olives

1-2 tbsp dressing made with extra-virgin olive oil, sesame, walnut or rapeseed oil

Toasted seeds or nuts: pumpkin, sunflower, pine nuts, hazelnuts, cashews

1-2 portions of pulses, squash or wholegrains, such as:

50g cooked quinoa, brown rice, whole barley or wild red rice

1 slice wholegrain bread: millet, spelt or rye (or gluten-free as required)

50g cooked beans, lentils or chickpeas

100g diced pumpkin or butternut squash

And for extra flavour:

Fermented vegetables, such as sauerkraut or kimchi

Pickled vegetables, such as cornichons, jalapeño peppers, olives

Seaweed: nori cut into strips, kelp/dulse flakes

Fresh herbs: coriander, mint, parsley, basil, etc

PHYTONUTRIENTS, also known as phytochemicals, are concentrated in the skins of fruits and vegetables and are responsible for their colour, scent and flavour. The best-known phytonutrients are carotenoids and flavonoids (found in yellow, orange, red, blue and purple fruit and vegetables), and polyphenols (found in foods like cocoa, olives, tea, coffee and red wine).

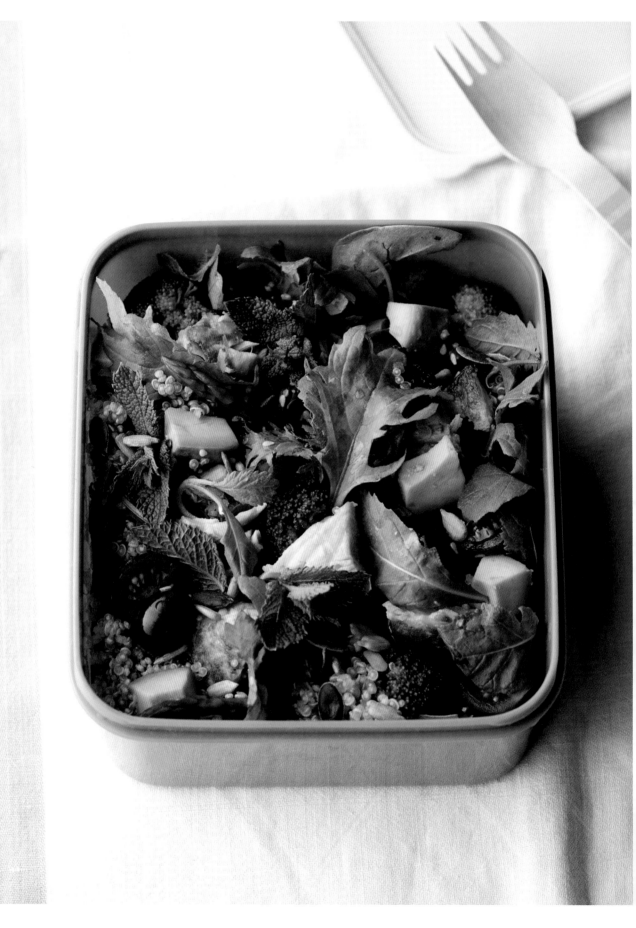

Phyto Salad Lunchbox with Salmon and Avocado

Serves 1

1. Colours:

4 asparagus spears, steamed

½ red pepper, deseeded and sliced

5 baby tomatoes, halved

2. Greens:

Small handful of mixed leaves

4-5 broccoli florets, steamed

3. Proteins:

125g salmon fillet, grilled

2 tbsp mixed seeds, toasted

4. Health-boosting fats:

½ avocado, sliced

6 olives

5. Optional wholegrains or squash:

50g cooked red and white quinoa or 50g roasted squash

And for extra flavour:

Kefir Mustard Dressing (page 119)

Handful of fresh mint, chopped

Maldon sea salt and pepper

• DAIRY-FREE OPTION

• GLUTEN-FREE OPTION

• GOOD FOR PHASE 1

1. In a large bowl, or a Tupperware box if you're taking it to work, toss together the sliced asparagus, red pepper, tomatoes, mixed leaves, broccoli, avocado, olives and quinoa.

2. Next add the salmon, and scatter the seeds and mint on top.

3. Make the dressing and put it in a small screw-top jar (if you're taking it to work).

4. When you're ready to eat, pour over the dressing and toss everything together.

730 CALORIES

Chinese Noodle Jar

Posh pot noodles to take to work – all you need is a spoon and some boiling water. In this recipe you can substitute the tofu with prawns or diced chicken and add different crunchy vegetables.

Serves 1

50g wholegrain soba noodles, cooked and cooled

150g chopped veg, such as broccoli, pak choi, spring greens, mange touts, mushrooms, bean sprouts

60g edamame beans

1 small spring onion, trimmed and sliced

30g cashew nuts

80g firm tofu, cubed

Small handful of fresh coriander, chopped

For the sauce:

2 tsp tamari sauce

1 tsp miso paste or ½ vegetable stock cube

½cm root ginger, grated

¼ tsp red chilli, diced

½ tsp sesame oil

2 tsp rice vinegar or apple cider vinegar

You will also need:

500ml jar with screw-top lid, or Kilner jar

1 small plastic container with a tight-fitting lid, for the sauce

•DAIRY-FREE

•GLUTEN-FREE

•GOOD FOR PHASE 1

1. Place the noodles, vegetables, beans, spring onion, cashews, tofu and coriander in the jar in layers so that it is about three-quarters full, and put the lid on.

2. Mix together the sauce ingredients in a small plastic container and put the lid on.

3. When you are ready to eat, add 50ml hot water to the sauce to loosen it and pour it into the jar, along with 200-250ml boiling water. Push the vegetables down into the water and give it all a stir, then allow it to rest for 4-5 minutes. Eat the mixture directly from the jar or tip it into a bowl.

Tips: make up extra portions of sauce and keep it in the fridge to use later in the week. You can use other noodles, such as rice noodles, glass noodles (these don't need cooking) or konjac noodles which are seriously low-carb.

300 CALORIES

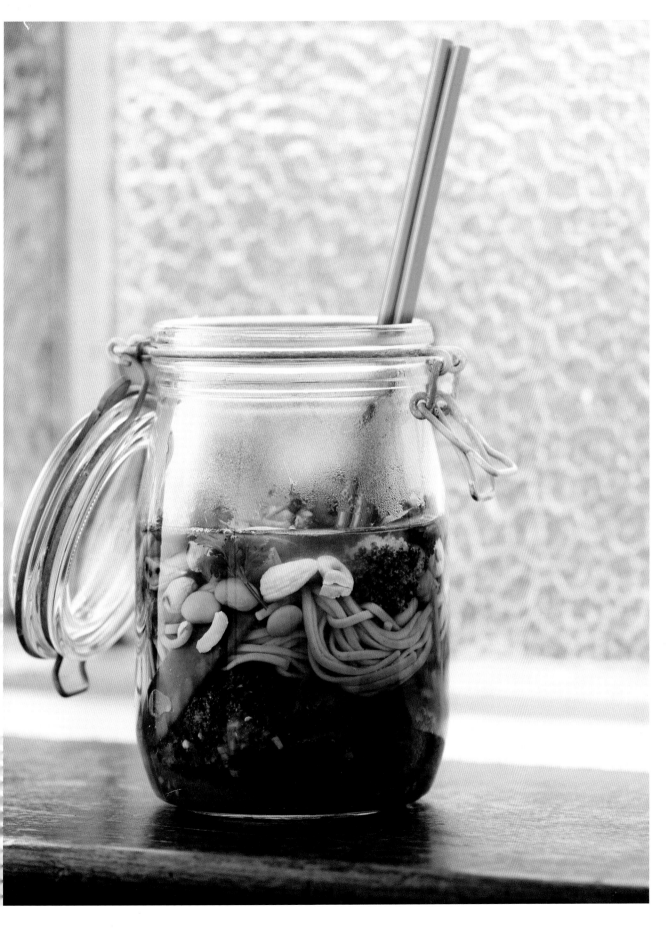

Beetroot and Yoghurt Dip

This vibrant purple dip has a hint of North Africa and is delicious as an accompaniment to a salad or as a colourful side dish.

Serves 4 as a side dish

400g beetroot, scrubbed
  and quartered
4 tbsp olive oil
2 large garlic cloves,
  finely diced
1 tsp ground cumin
½ tsp ground coriander
150g full-fat live Greek-
  style yoghurt (or non-
  dairy equivalent)
2 tsp capers, drained
  and rinsed

•DAIRY-FREE OPTION
•GLUTEN-FREE
•GOOD FOR PHASE 1

1. Preheat the oven to 180°C/160°C fan/gas mark 4. Toss the beetroots with the oil, garlic, cumin and coriander in a roasting tin and roast them until they are tender, around 40-50 minutes.

2. Allow them to cool slightly, then blend them in a food processor with the yoghurt and capers until they are well combined but still have a bit of texture.

3. Season the dip with sea salt and black pepper. Serve it with vegetable crudités, Flaxseed Crackers (page 78) or Wholemeal Flatbread (page 195).

200 CALORIES

Chargrilled Red Pepper Dip

Chickpeas can moderate your glucose metabolism, and contain resistant starches which produce short-chain fatty acids important for colon health. Even IBS sufferers can usually tolerate them.

Serves 6 as a dip
(2-4 as a side dish)

2 medium red peppers,
   halved and deseeded
   (or about 100g chargrilled
   red peppers from a jar,
   drained)
400g can chickpeas,
   drained
5 tbsp extra-virgin olive oil
1 tsp salt
1 garlic clove, crushed
Grated zest and juice
   of ½ lemon
Handful of fresh coriander,
   chopped
½ tsp chilli flakes to taste
Large pinch of paprika
   to serve

• DAIRY-FREE
• GLUTEN-FREE
• GOOD FOR PHASE 1

1. Place the pepper halves under a hot grill, skin side up, or over a flame until the skin has charred. Put them in a resealable bag to let them sweat, which helps to loosen the skin. Once they have cooled, remove the skin and place them in a food processor with the remaining ingredients.

2. Blitz until you have a smooth paste.

3. Serve the dip drizzled with a little olive oil and a sprinkling of paprika and some vegetable crudités on the side.

Tip: you can substitute the chickpeas with butterbeans, though these can exacerbate IBS symptoms in some people so are probably best avoided and only added in Phase 2. Like chickpeas, they are rich in protein, fibre, iron and B vitamins.

160 CALORIES

Lemon and Coriander Hummus with Seaweed

Tahini paste is made from ground sesame seeds, and combined with chickpeas provides an ideal balance of amino acids for protein absorption. The seaweed adds lovely marine omega 3.

Serves 6

400g can chickpeas, drained and rinsed

1 large garlic clove

1 level tbsp tahini

2 tbsp full-fat live Greek-style yoghurt (or non-dairy equivalent)

1 tbsp Preserved Lemons (page 184), seeds removed (or zest and juice of 1 lemon)

3 tbsp olive oil

1 nori seaweed sheet, finely sliced, plus a little extra for garnish

Large handful of coriander, including stalks, chopped

• DAIRY-FREE OPTION

• GLUTEN-FREE

• GOOD FOR PHASE 1

1. Blitz all the ingredients apart from the coriander in a food processor, leaving a bit of texture. Add the coriander and pulse briefly.

2. Leave it to rest for 30 minutes to bring out the flavours if time permits, then drizzle with olive oil and garnish with a few slices of chopped seaweed before serving.

140 CALORIES

Avocado and Lime Salsa

Creamy, tangy and slightly piquant, this makes a brilliant dip or accompaniment to a meal. It is full of nutrients and natural fats.

Serves 2

1 avocado, diced

½ red onion, finely diced

½-1 tsp chilli flakes to taste

1 tbsp fresh coriander or
   basil, chopped

1 tbsp lime juice

½ tbsp olive oil

• DAIRY-FREE

• GLUTEN-FREE

• GOOD FOR PHASE 1

1. Place all the ingredients except the olive oil in a dish and mash them together. Season with Maldon sea salt and freshly ground black pepper and drizzle over the olive oil.

2. Serve the salsa as a dip with vegetable crudités, or as a side dish with fish.

Smoked Mackerel Pâté

Mouth-watering, quick to make and full of essential omega 3 fats.

Serves 4

150g smoked mackerel
   fillets, skinned

3 tbsp full-fat live Greek-
   style yoghurt (or non-
   dairy equivalent)

1 tsp creamed horseradish

Juice of 1 lemon

• DAIRY-FREE OPTION

• GLUTEN-FREE

• GOOD FOR PHASE 1

1. Flake the fish into a dish, add the remaining ingredients and mix everything together well. Season with freshly ground black pepper.

2. Serve it with Flaxseed Crackers (page 78) or Thai Flavoured Seaweed Crackers (page 79), or spread it on Spinach and Ricotta Blinis (page 80).

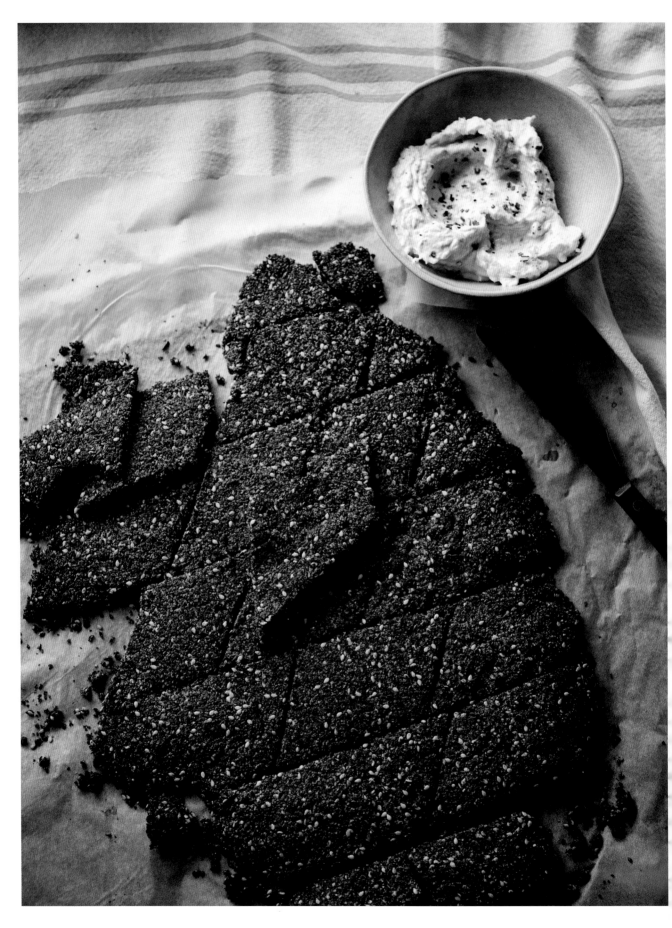

3 Cream Cheese Spreads

Dairy is thankfully no longer seen as one of the major causes of cardiovascular disease and diabetes. In fact, recent research suggests that it may even have a beneficial effect on these conditions. It's also a great source of calcium and protein. These spreads taste great served on rye bread, our Flaxseed Crackers (see page 78; shown left, with Horseradish Spread) or simply on finely sliced, toasted wholemeal soda bread.

Each serves 2

Horseradish

140g full-fat soft cheese
2 tsp creamed horseradish
1 tsp rosemary leaves,
   finely chopped

Mix the ingredients together in a bowl and serve as a dip or spread. You might top it with some pickled herring.

190 CALORIES

Smoked Salmon

140g full-fat soft cheese
60g smoked salmon, diced
Juice of ½ lemon
Small handful of dill,
   chopped
Generous grinding of black
   pepper

Mix the ingredients together in a bowl and serve as a dip or spread.

240 CALORIES

Beetroot and Chilli

140g full-fat soft cheese
100g cooked beetroot,
   diced
2 tsp chives, chopped
1 tsp lemon juice
Pinch of chilli flakes

•ALL GLUTEN-FREE

Blend the cream cheese with half the beetroot, the chives, lemon juice and chilli flakes in a small food processor until smooth. Stir in the remaining beetroot and serve sprinkled with freshly ground black pepper.

210 CALORIES

Flaxseed Crackers

Flaxseed is fast becoming another popular 'super food', packed as it is with protein, omega 3, vitamins and minerals. These crackers also contain lignans, which have strong antioxidant properties, and may help prevent some common cancers.

Makes about 20 crackers
200g ground flaxseeds
50g sesame seeds
2 tbsp chia seeds
1 tsp Marmite (or 1 tbsp vegan yeast if you're gluten-sensitive)
½ tsp Maldon sea salt

• DAIRY-FREE
• GLUTEN-FREE OPTION
• GOOD FOR PHASE 1

1. Preheat the oven to 120°C/100°C fan/gas mark ½. Place the flaxseeds, sesame seeds and chia seeds in a bowl.

2. Dissolve the Marmite in 50ml boiling water, then add 100ml cold water. Pour it into the seed mixture and stir vigorously until you have a gloopy paste. If it is dry or crumbly, add a little more water. Leave it to firm up for about 10 minutes.

3. Spread the mixture on baking paper or a silicone baking sheet. Place another piece of baking paper on top and use a rolling pin to flatten it to approximately 3-4mm thickness. Remove the top piece of baking paper and lightly score the surface so the dough can be separated into 20 square crackers. Scatter the salt over it.

4. Bake the dough in the middle of the oven for 30-40 minutes, until it is just starting to turn golden brown around the edges. Check it frequently, as it will taste bitter if you overcook it. Turn it over, then turn off the oven and leave it to dry out for at least 30 minutes. Once it has cooled, break it up into squares. The crackers will keep for up to 5 days in an airtight container.

Tip: if using vegan yeast, add it to the bowl with the seeds before adding the water.

80 CALORIES PER CRACKER

Thai-Flavoured Seaweed Crackers

These irresistibly moreish gluten-free crackers are high in fibre and give a good seaweed boost. You and your biome will love them. Try them with a dip, crumbled into a soup, or simply savour them on their own.

Makes about 24 crackers
100g buckwheat flour
100g ground flaxseeds
50g sesame seeds
2 nori seaweed sheets,
  chopped
½ tsp chilli flakes (optional)
1 tbsp Thai fish sauce
2 tbsp tamari sauce
1 tsp sesame oil

•DAIRY-FREE
•GLUTEN-FREE
•GOOD FOR PHASE 1

1. Preheat the oven to 120°C/100°C fan/gas mark ½. Place the flour, flaxseeds, sesame seeds, nori and chilli flakes, if using, in a bowl.

2. Add 3-4 tbsp water along with the Thai fish sauce and tamari sauce and stir vigorously to produce a very wet, sticky dough. If it is dry or crumbly, add more water gradually. Leave it to rest and firm up for about 10 minutes.

3. Spread the mixture on baking paper or a silicone baking sheet lightly greased with sesame oil. Place another greased piece of baking paper on top and use a rolling pin to roll it to approximately 3-4mm thickness. Remove the top piece of baking paper and lightly score the surface so the dough can be separated into 24 square crackers.

4. Bake the dough in the middle of the oven for 30-40 minutes, until it is just starting to turn golden brown around the edges. Check it frequently, as it will taste bitter if overcooked. Turn it over, then turn off the oven and leave it to dry out for at least 30 minutes. Let it cool completely on a wire rack before breaking it up into squares. The crackers will keep for up to 5 days in an airtight container.

160 CALORIES PER CRACKER

Spinach and Ricotta Blinis

Delicious green blinis that are packed with nutrients and work brilliantly with our spreads (pages 77) and dips (pages 72-73). They can be included in Phase 1 as cheese tends to be better tolerated than milk and the quantity in each blini is small, but best avoid them if you are dairy-intolerant.

Makes about 8-10

150g fresh spinach (or
   frozen spinach defrosted
   and drained)
60g wholemeal buckwheat
   flour
1 tsp baking powder
25g Parmesan, grated
2 eggs
100g ricotta
2-3 tbsp milk (or non-dairy
   equivalent)
2 tbsp olive oil

•GLUTEN-FREE
•GOOD FOR PHASE 1

1. Place the spinach in a colander and pour over a kettle of boiling water, then refresh it under a cold running tap. Drain it well and squeeze out as much water as possible before chopping it finely.

2. Mix the flour, baking powder and Parmesan in a bowl with some seasoning.

3. Beat together the eggs and ricotta and pour them into the flour mixture, whisking in enough milk to produce a thick batter. Then stir in the chopped spinach.

4. Heat the oil in a large frying pan and cook the blinis in batches of 3 or 4, using a dessertspoonful of the mixture for each one. Cook them until they are golden brown, about 3-4 minutes on each side, then place them on kitchen paper to drain.

Tip: these are delicious topped with smoked salmon, a squeeze of lemon and some freshly ground black pepper.

120 CALORIES PER BLINI

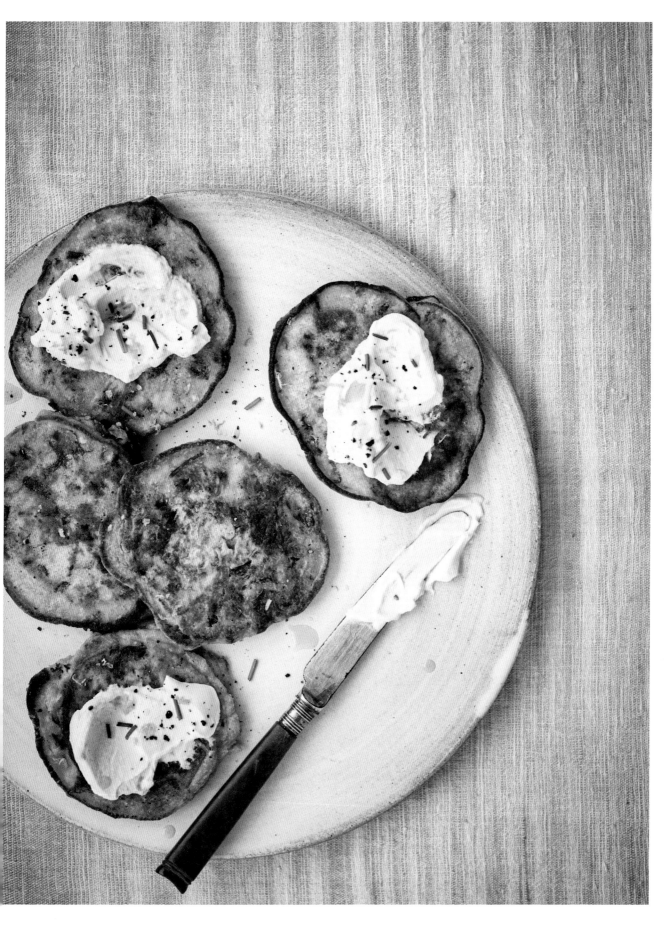

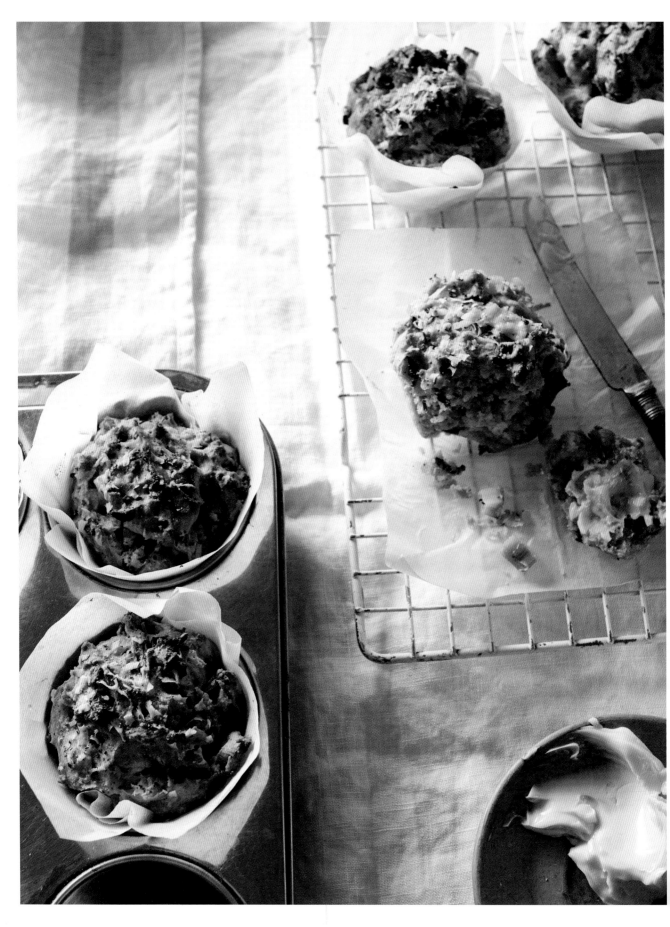

Sour Cream and Seaweed Muffins

Put one of these in your bag as you leave home. A tasty, nutritious snack to keep you from temptation...

Makes 12
50g butter, softened
4 spring onions, trimmed
  and finely chopped
2 large eggs
150ml buttermilk
160g sour cream and chive
  dip
1½ sheets nori seaweed,
  finely chopped
260g wholegrain flour, such
  as buckwheat or spelt
4 tbsp Parmesan, grated
1 tsp baking powder

•GLUTEN-FREE
•GOOD FOR PHASE 1

1. Preheat the oven to 180°C/160°C fan/gas mark 4. Line a 12-hole muffin tray with paper cases.

2. Melt the butter in a small frying pan and cook the spring onions for 3-4 minutes. In a bowl, beat together the eggs, buttermilk and sour cream dip, then stir in the cooked spring onions and the seaweed.

3. In a separate bowl, mix together the flour, Parmesan and baking powder and season with salt and plenty of freshly ground black pepper. Make a well in the centre of the dry ingredients and pour in the egg mixture. Combine everything well, but take care not to overmix.

4. Spoon the mixture into the muffin cases and bake for 18-20 minutes or until the tops are golden. They taste good hot or cold.

Tip: these muffins freeze well.

200 CALORIES EACH

Smoked Salmon Ceviche

This mildly exotic-tasting oily fish salad is ideal for a fasting-day lunch. Smoked salmon is remarkably filling yet low in calories. You also get some added protein, nutrients and fibre from the edamame beans.

Serves 1

Juice of 1 lime (or ½-1 tbsp yuzu juice)

1 tbsp live organic apple cider vinegar

½ tsp mirin wine (or ¼ tsp sugar)

¼ tsp root ginger, finely grated

Pinch of cayenne pepper or mild chilli powder

60g smoked salmon, diced

40g edamame beans, cooked

2-3 radishes, finely sliced

40g watercress

½ avocado, diced

1 tbsp mild olive oil

• DAIRY-FREE
• GLUTEN-FREE
• GOOD FOR PHASE 1

1. Mix the lime juice, cider vinegar, mirin, ginger and cayenne pepper in a bowl. Stir in the salmon, edamame beans and radishes and leave the mixture to marinate for 30 minutes.

2. When you are ready to eat, toss the watercress and avocado in the olive oil in another bowl and place the salmon mixture on top.

Tips: diced off-cuts of smoked salmon work fine and are far cheaper. Alternatively use 150g good-quality fillet of salmon cut into small cubes. Yuzu juice is a Japanese citrus fruit with a particularly tangy and sharp flavour – it is available in some supermarkets.

450 CALORIES

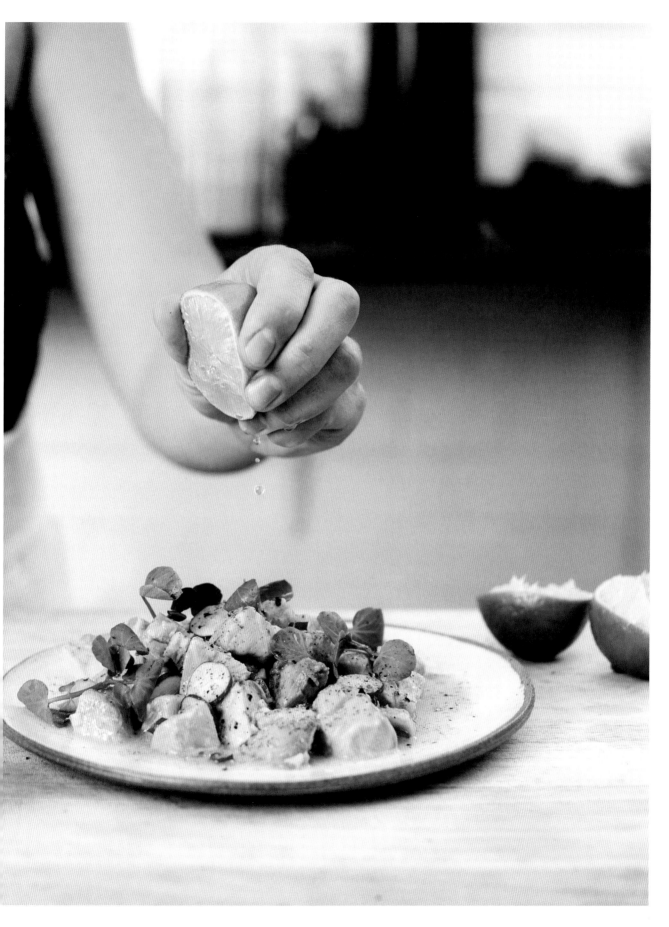

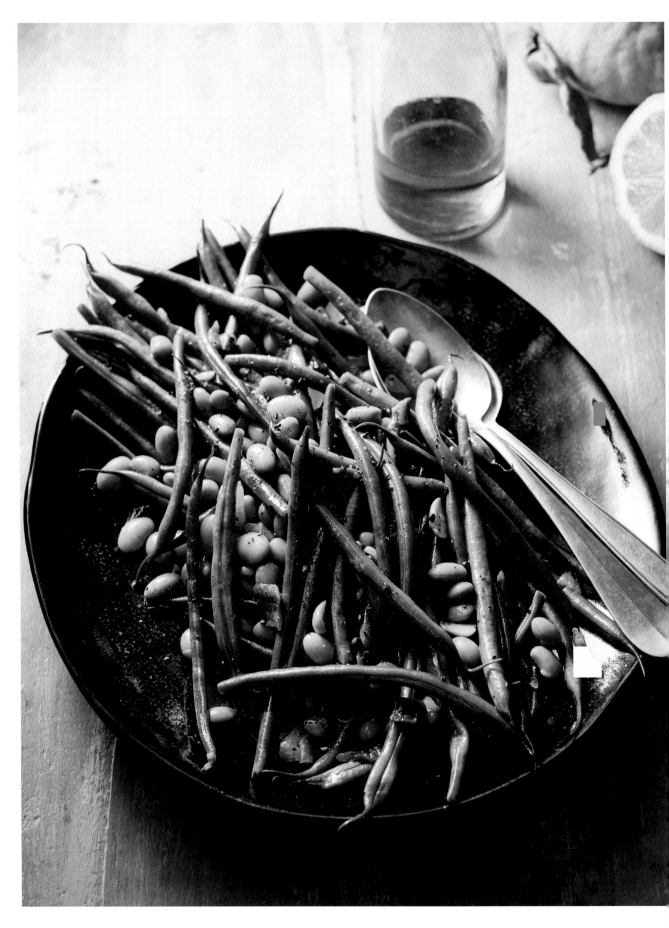

Green Beans and Edamame with Anchovies

This salad contains a good amount of protein and plenty of fibre to nourish your microbiome.

Serves 2

8 salted anchovies, rinsed
   and chopped
Juice of ½ lemon
2 tbsp olive oil
100g frozen edamame
   beans
150g thin green beans,
   topped and tailed

• DAIRY-FREE
• GLUTEN-FREE

1. Mix the anchovies with the lemon juice and olive oil in a medium-sized bowl.

2. Bring a pan of salted water to the boil and add the frozen edamame beans. Bring it back to the boil before adding the green beans, then simmer for 3-4 minutes, until the beans are al dente. Drain them, then stir them into the anchovy mixture. Add a generous grinding of black pepper and serve.

Note: in Phase 1 you may wish to reduce your portion size as the 'scratchy' fibres in both beans can exacerbate IBS.

240 CALORIES

Warm Lentil Salad

Serves 2

150g Puy lentils, rinsed well
1 garlic clove
1 bay leaf
1 red onion, finely chopped
3 medium tomatoes,
   chopped
50g spinach
1 tbsp balsamic vinegar
2 tbsp extra-virgin olive oil
75g goat's cheese (or non-
   dairy cheese), chopped
Handful of fresh parsley,
   chopped

• DAIRY-FREE OPTION
• GLUTEN-FREE

1. Place the lentils in a saucepan with the garlic, bay leaf and 2 cups of cold water. Bring it to the boil and simmer gently for 20 minutes, or until the lentils are tender.

2. Drain the lentils, discarding the garlic and bay leaf, and leave them to cool for 5 minutes in a salad bowl.

3. Stir the remaining ingredients into the warm lentils, season well with salt and freshly ground black pepper and sprinkle with parsley to serve.

Note: lentils can make IBS worse. Reduce or avoid in Phase 1.

440 CALORIES

Terra Mare Salad with Marine Phukka

This salad is so nutritious it's hard to know where to start. In fact, it may be the most gut-friendly recipe in this book… It has diverse dietary fibres from both sea and land, as well as other important metabolites, linked to gut health. It was given to us by marine conservationist and sustainable seaweed producer, Dr Pia Winberg.

Serves 2

80g quinoa

4 tbsp olive oil

2 leeks, diced

200g squid (fresh or frozen)

20-30g Phukka seaweed dukkah (or another dukkah blend)

1 lemon, ½ for juice and ½ cut into wedges

Rocket and baby spinach leaves

•DAIRY-FREE

•GLUTEN-FREE

•GOOD FOR PHASE 1

1. Rinse the quinoa well and cook it according to the pack instructions.

2. Heat 2 tbsp oil in a frying pan and sauté the leek gently for 6-8 minutes.

3. Meanwhile, cut open the squid, lay it flat with the inside facing up and criss-cross the surface with a sharp knife. Slice it into 1cm strips.

4. In another frying pan, heat the remaining oil and stir-fry the squid for a couple of minutes, taking care not to overcook it or it will be rubbery.

5. Remove it from the heat and toss it in the Phukka, the lemon juice and some salt and pepper. Mix it in a large bowl with the quinoa, leeks, rocket and baby spinach, and serve it with the lemon wedges.

400 CALORIES

SEAWEEDS have uniquely high levels of soluble dietary fibres (over 25% of their dry weight) and provide one of the best sources of the anti-ionflammatory omega-3 fatty acids. Studies have shown that the type of seaweed used in this Dukkah blend increases specific bacteria in the gut that are known to protect the mucous lining, as well as reduce inflammation.

Toasted Slaw with Halloumi and Lemony Buttermilk Dressing

The purple broccoli and red cabbage in this dish boost your phytonutrient intake and the buttermilk dressing tops up your probiotics. By heating and slightly toasting the crisper vegetables you make them easier to digest.

Serves 2

100g red cabbage leaves, finely sliced

100g green cabbage leaves, finely sliced

100g purple sprouting broccoli, cut into bite-sized pieces

2 tbsp olive oil

50g shiitaki or chestnut mushrooms, sliced

150g halloumi, sliced

Generous handful of bitter salad leaves (spinach, rocket or dandelion)

½ portion of Lemony Buttermilk Dressing (page 118)

1 tbsp flaked almonds, toasted

•GLUTEN-FREE

1. Scorch the cabbage and broccoli slices on a very hot griddle, turning them once. This should take about 2 minutes on each side. Then tip them into a wide salad bowl.

2. Meanwhile, heat the olive oil in a frying pan and fry the mushrooms and halloumi slices until they are golden, then stir them into the cabbage mixture.

3. Add the salad leaves and toss everything in the Lemony Buttermilk Dressing. Sprinkle the toasted almonds on top before serving.

530 CALS WITH DRESSING

Warm Red Rice Salad with Courgettes

Serves 2

120g precooked red
   Camargue rice
2 courgettes, sliced
¼ small cabbage, sliced
40g pine nuts, toasted
1 tbsp Preserved Lemons,
   diced (page 184)
Juice of 1 lemon
2 tbsp extra-virgin olive oil
2 tbsp fresh parsley,
   chopped
1 tsp fresh mint, chopped
2 tsp fresh thyme, chopped

•DAIRY-FREE
•GLUTEN-FREE
•GOOD FOR PHASE 1

1. Reheat the rice by adding 1 tbsp water and placing it in a microwave or steaming it in a pan. Then spoon it into a salad bowl.

2. Place the courgette slices and cabbage on a very hot griddle for a couple of minutes, turning them as they char. Stir them into the rice, along with the rest of the ingredients.

Tip: if you don't have preserved lemons, you can use the grated zest of 1 lemon.

370 CALORIES

Broccoli and Asparagus with Buttermilk Dressing

Serves 2

¼ head of broccoli
¼ cauliflower
300g asparagus, tips only
2 tbsp pumpkin seeds
1 cos lettuce, sliced
¼ red onion, finely sliced
100g feta, crumbled
½ portion of Turmeric
   Buttermilk Dressing
   (page 119)

•GLUTEN-FREE

1. Break the cauliflower and broccoli into florets and place them on a hot griddle for 3-4 minutes, turning them as they char. Tip them into a wide serving bowl, then cook the asparagus in the same way.

2. Toast the pumpkin seeds in a small pan until they start to pop, then remove them from the heat.

3. Once the veg have cooled a bit, add the lettuce and onion and toss everything in the dressing. Scatter the feta and pumpkin seeds on top.

360 CALORIES

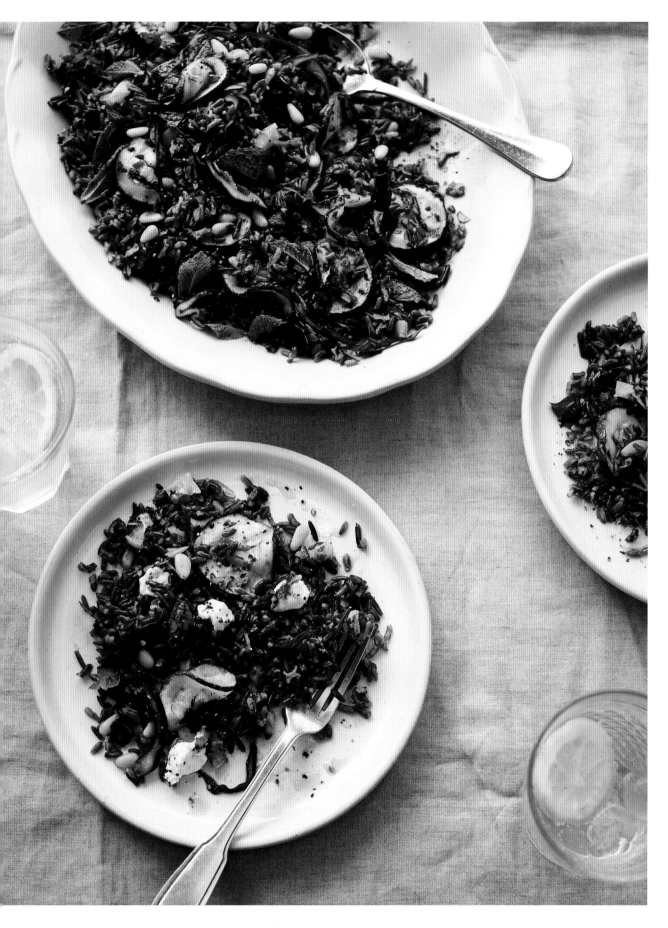

Low-Carb Mac 'n' Cheese

Macaroni cheese is experiencing a renaissance, a classic home-cooked comfort food that it is now being served in top restaurants. Here is a relatively low-carb version that is creamy, nutritious and satisfying, with a mild chilli kick.

Serves 2

80g green-pea macaroni twists (or gluten-free wholemeal macaroni)

75g cauliflower florets

60g broccoli florets

2 tbsp olive oil

1 garlic clove, crushed

½-1 green jalapeño chilli from a jar, diced

100g mature Cheddar cheese

150g full-fat crème fraîche

25g Parmesan, grated

•GLUTEN-FREE

1. Preheat the oven to 180°C/160°C fan/gas mark 4. Boil the pasta according to the pack instructions. Drain it when it is al dente and rinse it under cold running water.

2. Toss the cauliflower and broccoli florets in the olive oil and a generous pinch of salt, then spread them out on a baking tray or in a roasting tin. Bake them for 10-15 minutes or until they start to brown around the edges, then transfer them to a medium-sized baking dish. Stir in the pasta with the garlic and chilli.

3. In a bowl, mix together the Cheddar and crème fraîche. Spread this mixture on top of the vegetables, followed by a sprinkling of Parmesan and freshly ground black pepper.

4. Bake it in the oven for 12-15 minutes or until the top is turning golden brown and the cheesy sauce is bubbling.

Tip: this is delicious served with Green Beans and Edamame with Anchovies (page 87).

750 CALORIES

Kale and Tofu Scramble

A spicy vegan alternative to scrambled eggs. Very tasty it is too.

Serves 2

3 tbsp olive oil

1 tsp cumin seeds

½ tsp paprika

240g firm tofu, chopped
into 1½-2cm pieces

250g cauliflower, broken
into florets

75g pine nuts

2 large handfuls of kale,
chopped, tough stalks
removed

2 tbsp fresh coriander,
chopped

• DAIRY-FREE
• GLUTEN-FREE
• GOOD FOR PHASE 1

1. Preheat the oven to 180°C/160°C fan/gas mark 4. In a bowl, mix together the oil, spices and some seasoning. Stir in the tofu, followed by the cauliflower.

2. Spread the mixture out in a roasting tin and bake it for 20 minutes, stirring it from time to time. Scatter the pine nuts on top 5 minutes before the end of cooking time.

3. Meanwhile, steam the kale until it's just tender, around 2-3 minutes, then divide it between 2 plates. Scatter the cauliflower and tofu mixture over the top, and finish with a sprinkling of chopped coriander.

Tip: instead of steaming the kale you can stir it into the roasting tin with the tofu and cauliflower when you add the pine nuts.

580 CALORIES

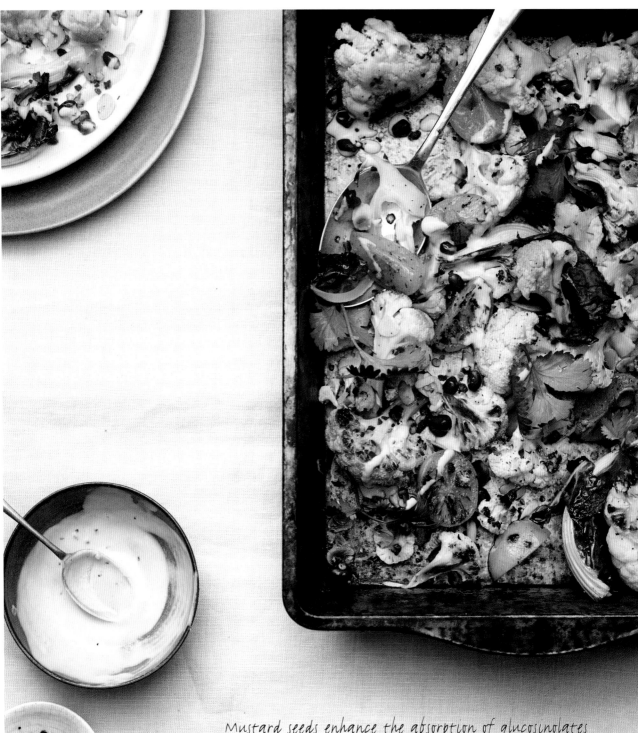

Mustard seeds enhance the absorption of glucosinolates from cruciferous vegetables such as cauliflower, cabbage, kale, Brussel sprouts and broccoli, which are thought to protect against inflammation and some cancers.

Cauliflower Baked with Lemon and Almonds

A scrumptious alternative to starchy potatoes, and one that your gut bacteria will love.

Serves 4

1 large cauliflower, cut
   into florets
4 tbsp extra-virgin olive oil
1 tbsp Preserved Lemons
   (page 184), or zest
   and juice of 1 lemon
1 tsp mustard seeds
50g flaked almonds
½ tsp chilli flakes
Juice of 1 lemon

• DAIRY-FREE
• GLUTEN-FREE
• GOOD FOR PHASE 1

1. Preheat the oven to 180°C/160°C fan/gas mark 4. Spread the florets in a large roasting tin.

2. Drizzle over the olive oil and season well with sea salt and freshly ground black pepper. Place the tray in the oven for 10 minutes.

3. Remove from the oven and mix in the preserved lemon and chilli, and scatter over the mustard seeds and almonds. Cook for another 10-12 minutes, or until the cauliflower is tender and browning in places. Transfer it to a serving dish and drizzle over the lemon juice before serving.

Tip: for added flavour you can whip up a tahini drizzle, with 2 tbsp tahini, 1 tbsp fresh lemon juice and 1 tbsp warm water, seasoned with salt and pepper (add 60 cals). And for a bit more crunch and colour you might scatter on some pomegranate seeds a few minutes before serving. (Avoid pomegranate during Phase 1 as its tough fibre can exacerbate IBS symptoms).

220 CALORIES

Aubergine Parmigiana

A delicious, Mediterranean-style bake. Aubergine contains antioxidants such as anthocyanin, a pigment that, among other things, can protect against cellular damage.

Serves 2

1 large aubergine, cut into
   1cm slices
4 tbsp olive oil
1 garlic clove, diced
2 tsp fresh oregano,
   chopped (or 1 tsp dried)
150ml passata
125g mozzarella (or non-
   dairy cheese), sliced
50g cherry tomatoes,
   halved
50g Parmesan (or vegan
   Parmesan), finely grated

• DAIRY-FREE OPTION
• GLUTEN-FREE
• GOOD FOR PHASE 1

1. Preheat the oven to 180°C/160°C fan/gas mark 4. Brush the aubergine slices on both sides with 3 tbsp of the olive oil, then brown them on a very hot griddle.

2. Stir the garlic and oregano into the passata and pour it into an ovenproof dish. Lay the aubergine slices on top, followed by the mozzarella and the cherry tomatoes. Drizzle over the remaining olive oil, and finish with a sprinkling of Parmesan.

3. Bake the Parmigiana for 14-15 minutes, or until the top is lightly golden. Serve it with a crisp green salad.

Tip: throw in a handful of pitted olives for extra flavour (add 20 cals).

580 CALORIES

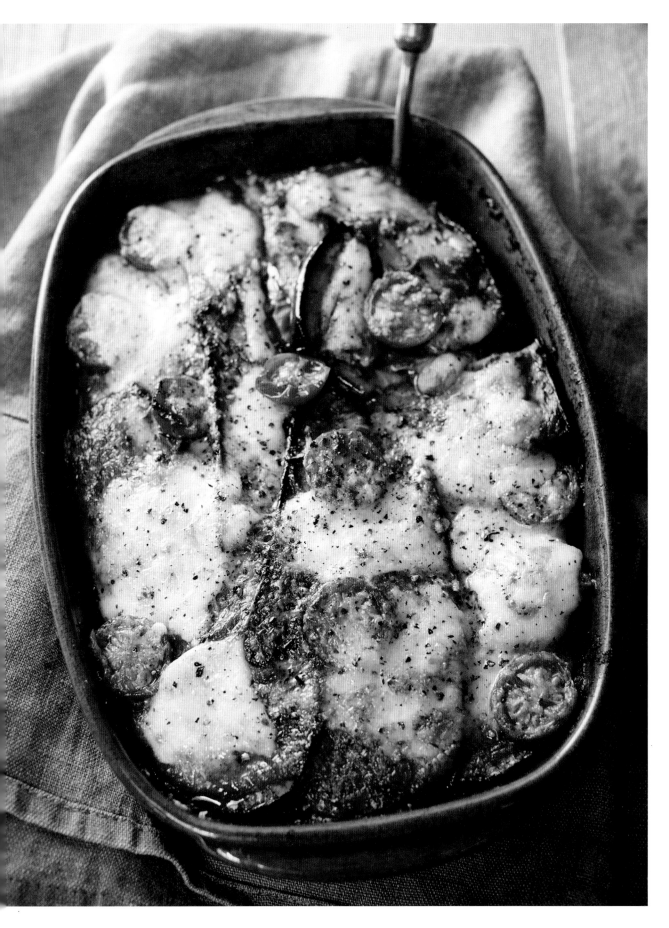

Michael's Mussels

A firm favourite in our household, and one that brings out the hunter-gatherer in Michael, who relishes scrubbing and preparing the mussels. Having said that, mussels are usually so well cleaned these days that there is hardly a tuft of seaweed beard left on them to remove. Mussels are probably the most sustainable source of high-quality protein you will find. Fiddly to eat, but worth it – savour their delicate, sweet and juicy flesh.

Serves 2

1kg fresh mussels in shells
2 tbsp olive oil
½ onion, finely diced
1 garlic clove, crushed
   or finely diced
125ml white wine
Sprig of fresh thyme
2 tbsp crème fraîche,
   (optional)
Generous handful of fresh
   parsley, chopped

•DAIRY-FREE OPTION
•GLUTEN-FREE
•GOOD FOR PHASE 1

1. Check each shell to make sure it closes when you tap it and scrub off any obvious chunks of seaweed. Discard any that remain open when tapped – the mussels need to be fresh and alive.

2. Sauté the onion in the olive oil in a large saucepan over a medium heat for about 5 minutes, adding the garlic after 3 minutes.

3. Pour in the wine, followed by the thyme and the mussels. Cover the pan with a well-fitting lid and bring it to the boil. Simmer gently for 4-5 minutes or until the mussels have opened. Discard any that remain shut.

4. Divide the mussels between 2 bowls, reserving the juices. Stir the crème fraîche (if using) and parsley into the juices before pouring them over the mussels. Serve them with chunks of fresh No-Knead Sourdough or Wholemeal Flatbread (pages 198 and 195) and a bitter leaf salad.

370 CALORIES

Pasta with Pistachio Pesto

Made with pistachio nuts, this rich creamy pesto has a gorgeous subtle flavour. You'll never want to go back to a shop-bought jar. Mixing spaghetti with some spiralised courgetti is a great pain-free way of reducing your carb consumption.

Serves 4

100g fresh basil

75g Parmesan (or vegan Parmesan), grated

120g pistachios

2 garlic cloves, chopped

150ml olive oil

4 medium courgettes or 300g butternut squash, spiralised

160g wholemeal spaghetti (or gluten-free alternative)

• DAIRY-FREE OPTION
• GLUTEN-FREE OPTION
• GOOD FOR PHASE 1

1. To make the pesto, blend the basil, Parmesan, pistachios and garlic in a food processor until they start to break down. Gradually add the olive oil until the mixture starts to thicken into a sauce. Season to taste.

2. Cook the spaghetti in salted water according to the pack instructions. Add the courgettes or butternut squash for the last minute of cooking. Drain the pasta and vegetables and tip them into a large serving bowl. Stir in the pesto so everything gets a good coating. Serve immediately.

Tip: if you buy 3 pots of basil from the supermarket and pinch off the large and medium leaves, leaving the small ones to grow, you will be able to make the pesto again in a few weeks' time.

580 CALORIES

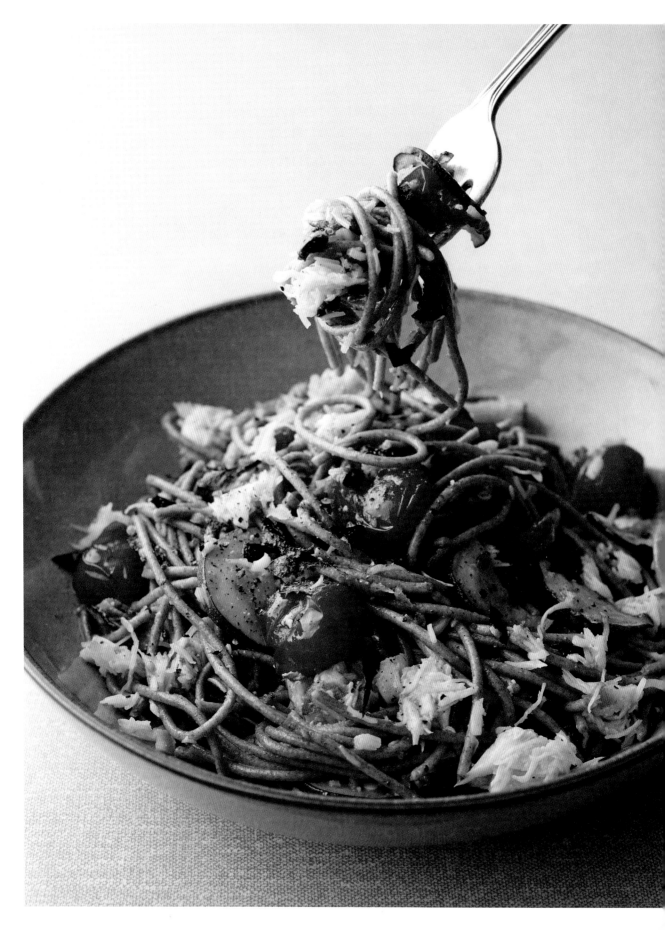

Crab Spaghetti with Seaweed

Crab is a great source of protein and selenium, which has anti-inflammatory properties. Its slightly sweet taste is enhanced here by the umami flavours of the seaweed.

Serves 2

300g wholegrain spaghetti or green-pea pasta (or gluten-free alternative)

3 tbsp olive oil

2-3 garlic cloves, finely chopped

1 red chilli, deseeded and finely chopped (or ½ tsp chilli flakes)

10 mini plum or cherry tomatoes

1 courgette, halved lengthways and sliced

200g crab meat (fresh, canned or frozen)

Juice of ½ large lemon

Large handful of fresh parsley, roughly chopped

1 nori seaweed sheet, chopped

• DAIRY-FREE
• GLUTEN-FREE OPTION
• GOOD FOR PHASE 1

1. Cook the pasta according to the pack instructions. Drain it when it is al dente, retaining 2 tbsp of the cooking water, then rinse it under cold running water and set it aside.

2. Meanwhile, heat the olive oil in a large frying pan and gently fry the garlic, chilli, tomatoes and courgette for 2-3 minutes. Stir in the crab meat and heat it through, then add the lemon juice.

3. Add the cooked pasta, along with the reserved cooking water, chopped parsley and nori. Stir well to warm the pasta through and ensure it gets a good even coating of the sauce. Season and serve with a dark-green leaf salad.

800 CALORIES

Poor Man's Potatoes with Anchovies

Based on a classic Spanish dish, *Papas a lo Pobre*, this makes a wonderfully comforting, easy meal.

Serves 4

400g baby new potatoes

5 tbsp olive oil

1 large red onion, finely sliced

1 large green pepper, deseeded and finely sliced

2 large garlic cloves, finely sliced

30g can anchovies, drained and chopped

Juice of ½ lemon

Sprig of rosemary or thyme

Large handful of fresh parsley, chopped

•DAIRY-FREE

•GLUTEN-FREE

•GOOD FOR PHASE 1

1. Ideally, use precooked potatoes, i.e. ones that have been boiled for 15-20 minutes in lightly salted water until they're tender, then cooled in the fridge for 12 hours to bring out the resistant starch. Otherwise, boil the potatoes and use them immediately.

2. Heat the olive oil in a large frying pan and sweat the onion and green pepper for 5 minutes before adding the potatoes, cut in half.

3. Add the garlic and cook for a further 1-2 minutes, then stir in the anchovies, lemon juice and thyme or rosemary sprig.

4. Simmer for 5 minutes, stirring occasionally, until the vegetables are tender but not browned. Season generously with black pepper and stir in the parsley. Serve with a multicoloured salad or other colourful vegetables.

Note: anyone with active IBS may need to reduce the amount of onions and garlic.

260 CALORIES

Green peppers are an excellent source of
vitamins A, C and B6. Anchovies
provide lots of lovely omega 3...

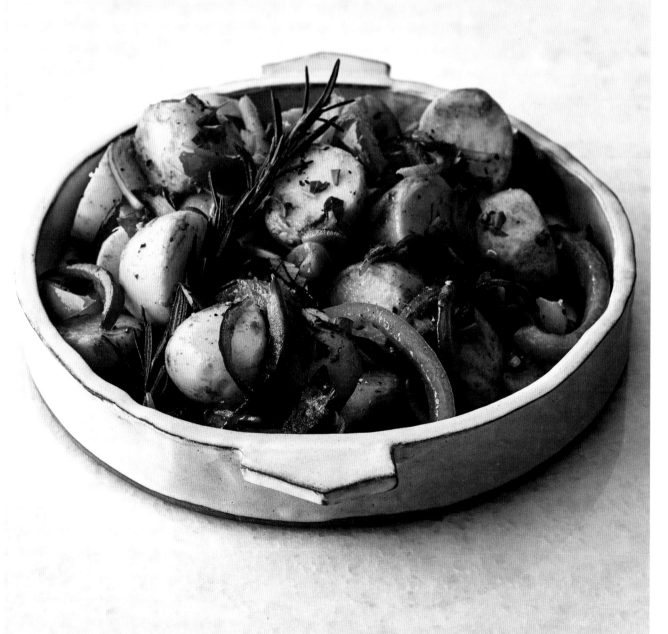

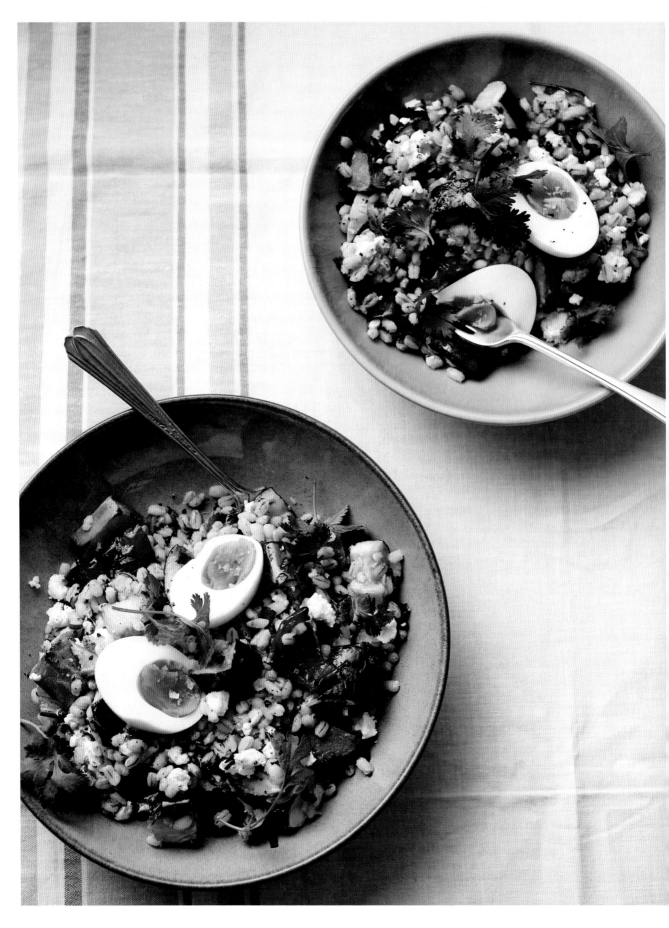

Roasted Mediterranean Vegetables, Pearl Barley and Eggs

If you haven't eaten pearl barley, here's a chance to try it out. Slow to release its starches, this delicious wholegrain provides a steady source of energy and delivers more fibre to feed your biome than the more processed grains. Can be eaten warm or cold.

Serves 2

1 small aubergine, diced

1 large courgette, sliced

1 red pepper, deseeded and sliced

125g butternut squash, deseeded and cubed

3 tbsp olive oil

100g pearl barley

2 eggs, hardboiled and cut into quarters

75g goat's cheese (or non-dairy cheese), crumbled

Handful of fresh parsley or coriander, chopped

Juice of ½ lemon

•DAIRY-FREE OPTION

•GOOD FOR PHASE 1

1. Preheat the oven to 200°C/180°C fan/gas mark 6. Place the aubergine, courgette, red pepper and butternut squash in a roasting tin and toss them in the olive oil and some seasoning.

2. Bake the vegetables for 30-40 minutes or until they're tender and browned at the edges, turning them once or twice.

3. Meanwhile, cook the pearl barley according to the pack instructions.

4. Remove the vegetables from the oven and stir in the pearl barley. Transfer everything to a serving dish, lightly stir in the eggs, and scatter the goat's cheese and parsley or coriander on top. Season to taste with Maldon sea salt, black pepper and lemon juice.

Tip: for a gluten-free version, swap the pearl barley for gluten-free bulgar wheat, quinoa or buckwheat. This is an ideal recipe for using up leftover grain, which of course contains extra gut-friendly resistant starch if it has been cooled in the fridge before being reheated.

520 CALORIES

Mackerel with Quinoa Tabbouleh

Of all the oily fish, mackerel has one of the highest concentrations of omega 3. Quinoa, meanwhile, is truly a miracle grain, containing thiamin, which helps create the digestive acids in your stomach; riboflavin, which is crucial for the health of the gut wall; and also amino acids such as glutamine, a primary source of energy for the gut, helping it produce adequate amounts of protective mucus – something that is particularly important during periods of strenuous exercise, stress or medical trauma.

Serves 4

225g quinoa

125g cooked beetroot, diced

1 carrot, grated

Large handful of fresh parsley, chopped

Large handful of fresh mint, chopped

Large handful of fresh coriander, chopped

Large handful of chives, chopped

1 tbsp pine nuts, lightly toasted

½ cucumber, diced

Juice of 1 lime

2 tbsp extra-virgin olive oil

4 large mackerel fillets

•DAIRY-FREE
•GLUTEN-FREE
•GOOD FOR PHASE 1

1. Cook the quinoa according to the pack instructions, then drain it and refresh it under cold running water. Put it in a large bowl and stir in the beetroot, carrot, herbs, pine nuts and cucumber. Add the lime juice, olive oil and some seasoning and mix everything together. Leave it to stand at room temperature while you cook the fish.

2. Season the mackerel fillets with salt and freshly ground black pepper, then grill them for 3-4 minutes on each side. Serve them on a bed of the tabbouleh.

Note: there has been some concern about the possible negative effect on the gut of the saponins that naturally coat and protect the quinoa seed. Just washing this layer off before use will eliminate the problem.

410 CALORIES

Chickpea, Coconut and Cashew Curry

A creamy vegetarian curry with plenty of flavour, but not too spicy. Chickpeas contain a moderate amount of carbohydrates. They are also a good source of fibre and protein.

Serves 2 as a main dish
(4 as a side dish)

3 tbsp mild olive oil
 or rapeseed oil
1 onion, diced
2 celery stalks, diced
1 garlic clove, diced
2cm root ginger, grated
 or finely diced
1 tsp ground cumin
1 tsp mustard seeds
1 tsp ground turmeric
400g can chickpeas,
 drained
200ml coconut milk
Juice of 1 lime
60g cashew nuts
Large handful of fresh
 coriander, chopped

• DAIRY-FREE
• GLUTEN-FREE
• GOOD FOR PHASE 1

1. Heat the oil in a pan and sauté the onion and celery for 4-5 minutes. Add the garlic, ginger and spices and cook for a further 2 minutes.

2. Stir in the chickpeas, followed by the coconut milk, lime juice and cashew nuts, and simmer for 15-20 minutes.

3. Stir in the coriander and some seasoning before serving. This curry is delicious with Warm Red Rice Salad with Courgettes (page 90).

Tip: to cook chickpeas from scratch, cover them in 8-10cm water and soak them overnight, then boil them in a partially covered pot with three times the volume of water. Simmer for about 1 1/2 hours or until they're tender, skimming off any foam on the surface.

710 CALORIES

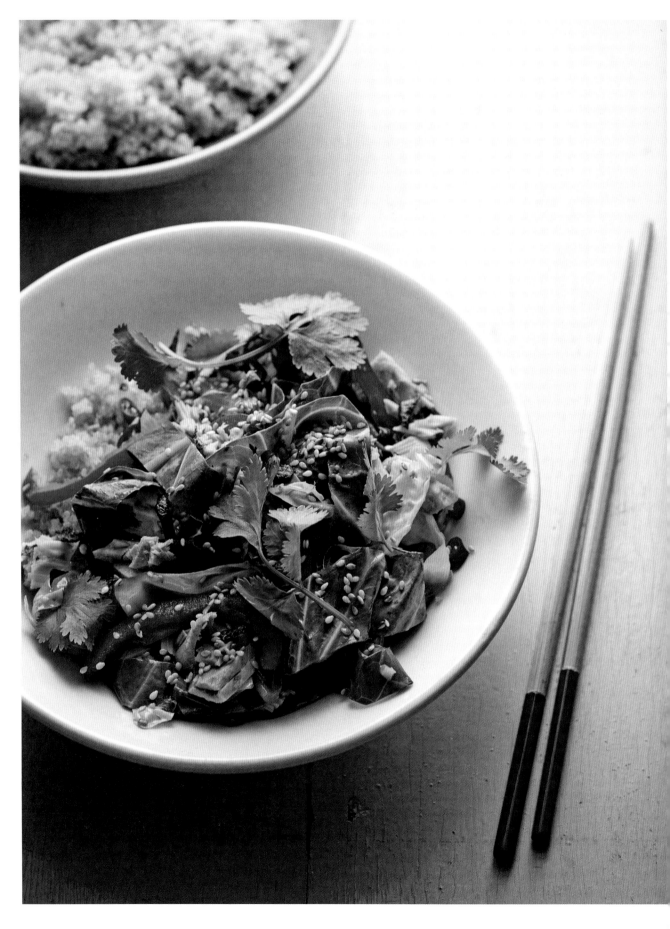

Tuna and Veg Stir-Fry with Seaweed

One of the easiest fish stir-fries you can make, conjured up with food from the store cupboard and veg you are likely to have in the fridge. What's more, it's bursting with omega 3 oils. We love it.

Serves 2

160g can tuna in oil, drained

1 tbsp fish sauce

1 tbsp rapeseed oil

1 small onion, sliced

1 red pepper, deseeded and chopped

2 celery stalks, sliced

100g spring greens or cabbage, shredded

1cm root ginger, diced

1 garlic clove, sliced

½ red chilli, deseeded and diced (or ¼ tsp chilli flakes)

1½ nori seaweed sheets, chopped or shredded

1 tbsp rice wine

• DAIRY-FREE
• GLUTEN-FREE
• GOOD FOR PHASE 1

1. Place the tuna in a bowl and sprinkle the fish sauce over it. Leave it to stand.

2. Heat the oil in a wok and stir-fry the onion, red pepper and celery for 3-4 minutes. Add the greens, ginger, garlic, chilli and nori and continue to stir-fry for 1-2 minutes. Reduce the heat and add the rice wine, along with 1-2 tbsp water.

3. Gently stir in the tuna, without breaking it up too much, and cook gently for a couple of minutes. Serve with Cauliflower Rice with Coriander (page 174) or 2 tbsp brown basmati rice (add 100 cals).

Note: you may need to reduce the amount of onion, garlic and red pepper if you have IBS.

Tip: to add flavour and texture scatter over 1-2 tsp toasted sesame seeds before serving.

580 CALORIES

Brazilian-Style Crab

Baked crab Brazilian-style, *Casquinha de Siri*, is a classic of the Bahia region where the cooking often involves an exotic combination of Mediterranean and African ingredients. Crab is rich in high-quality protein.

Serves 4

1 tbsp olive oil
½ small onion, finely
  chopped
1 large garlic clove,
  chopped
1 red pepper, deseeded
  and diced
250g white crab meat
  (fresh, canned or frozen)
2 medium tomatoes, peeled,
  deseeded and chopped
125ml coconut milk
Handful of fresh parsley,
  chopped
1 tbsp Parmesan (or vegan
  Parmesan), grated
Wedges of lime
Pinch of chilli flakes or
  a few drops of Tabasco
  sauce to serve

• DAIRY-FREE OPTION
• GLUTEN-FREE
• GOOD FOR PHASE 1

1. Preheat the oven to 180°C/160°C fan/gas mark 4. Heat the olive oil in a saucepan and sauté the onion for 5 minutes. Add the garlic and red pepper and cook for another 2-3 minutes, before adding the crab meat and tomatoes.

2. After 2 minutes, pour in the coconut milk and some seasoning and bring it to the boil. Stir in the parsley and transfer the mixture to a baking dish. Sprinkle the grated Parmesan on top, if using, and bake for 10-12 minutes, or until the top is golden.

3. Scatter over a few chilli flakes or drops of Tabasco, and serve it alongside a bitter leaf salad and some lime wedges.

370 CALORIES

Turmeric Coronation Chicken

An old favourite given a healthy twist. Turmeric has been shown to have an impact on reducing inflammation, and possibly even the risk of cancer. The fat in the creamy sauce and the generous amount of black pepper in this recipe will significantly increase the beneficial effects of the curcumin in the turmeric.

Serves 2

2 tbsp olive oil

1 small onion, diced

2 celery stalks, diced

30g dried apricots, diced

2 tsp ground turmeric

2 tsp curry powder

8 small cornichons, diced

1-2 tsp freshly ground
  black pepper

175g cooked chicken
  or turkey, chopped into
  bite-size pieces

125g full-fat live Greek-
  style yoghurt (or non-
  dairy equivalent)

75ml full-fat mayonnaise
  (or non-dairy equivalent)

Grated zest of 1 lime

2 tbsp fresh coriander,
  chopped

30g flaked almonds, toasted

•DAIRY-FREE OPTION

•GLUTEN-FREE

•GOOD FOR PHASE 1

1. Heat the olive oil in a pan and sauté the onion and celery for 4-5 minutes. Add the apricots and spices and cook for a further 2-3 minutes, then set the mixture aside to cool.

2. Stir in the cornichons, black pepper, chicken or turkey, yoghurt, mayonnaise, lime zest, most of the coriander and half of the nuts. Tip the mixture into a bowl, then scatter the remaining coriander and nuts on top.

3. Serve it with brown rice (for 2 tbsp add 100 cals), Cauliflower Rice with Coriander (page 174) or quinoa (for 2 tbsp add 120 cals) and a generous helping of bitter leaf salad such as rocket, watercress and/or baby spinach.

720 CALORIES

Spinach Dahl

This wonderful filling dahl can be eaten on its own or as a side dish. Full of creamy, rich coconut flavours, it reheats well so you can keep it for a second hit later in the week. Lentils are generally great for your microbiome, being highly nutritious and containing a fair amount of protein.

Serves 4 as a main dish,
(6-8 as a side dish)

3 tbsp olive oil or coconut oil

1 medium onion, chopped

2 garlic cloves, chopped

1 red chilli, deseeded and chopped (or ½ tsp chilli flakes)

1 tsp cumin seeds

1 tsp ground coriander

1 tsp ground turmeric

2cm root ginger, diced

Juice of ½ lemon

400ml can coconut milk

400g can green lentils, drained

100g spinach leaves (or kale, stalks removed)

1 tbsp fresh coriander, chopped

200g paneer, chopped into 2cm cubes (optional)

• DAIRY-FREE OPTION
• GLUTEN-FREE

1. Heat the oil in a medium-sized pan or casserole with a lid, and sauté the onion for 5 minutes. Stir in the garlic and cook for 1 more minute before adding the chilli, spices and ginger.

2. After 2 more minutes, stir in the lemon juice, coconut milk and lentils. Bring the pan to the boil, then put the lid on and allow it to simmer for 10 minutes, stirring occasionally and adding more water if needed.

3. Add the spinach (or kale) and cook for 3-5 minutes, then stir in the chopped coriander and season with salt and pepper. Scatter the paneer on top. You might serve this dahl with 1 tbsp Greek-style yoghurt (add 75 cals) and Onion and Courgette Bhajis (page 162).

Tips: instead of lentils, you can use yellow split peas (chana dahl), which take longer (35-40 minutes) to cook, or the smaller red lentils, which only take about 15 minutes, but give less texture. This dish freezes well and reheating it will increase the quantity of gut-friendly resistant starch too.

Note: if you have IBS, reduce your portion size as the lentils can exacerbate symptoms.

570 CALORIES

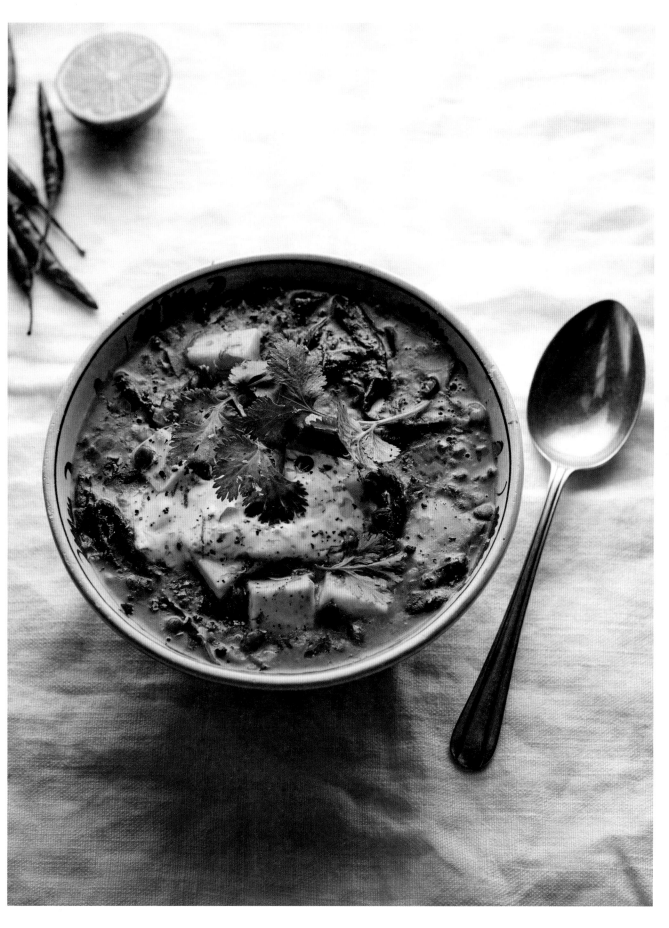

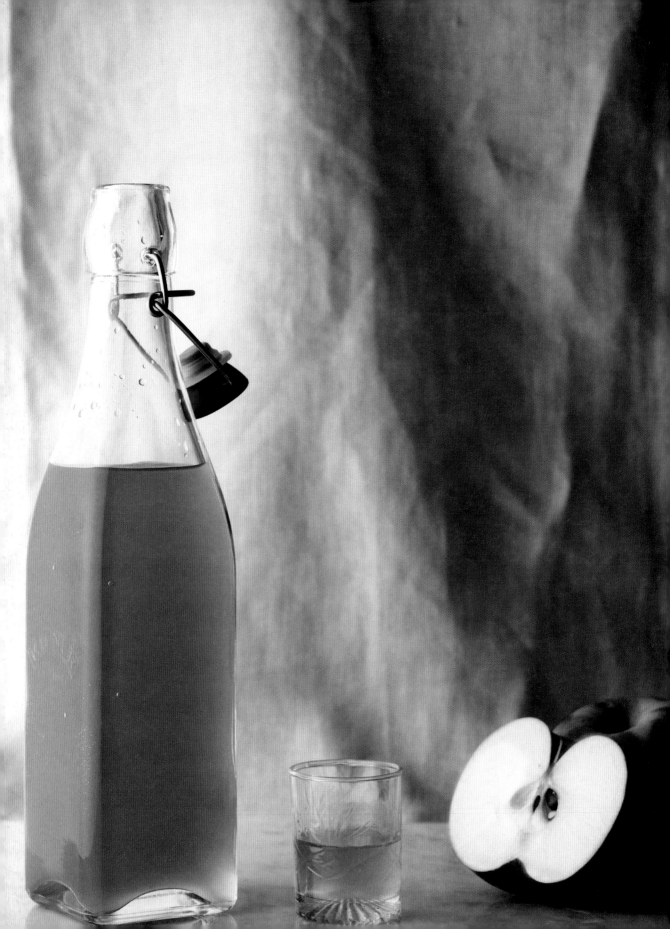

DRESSINGS AND FLAVOURINGS

Dressings tend to be considered an afterthought, but in this book we have brought them centre-stage. They will transform a dull salad, add zip to the simplest of vegetables and deliver lots of friendly bacteria to boost your biome...

Anchovy and Rosemary Dressing

Anchovy and rosemary make great companions in this lip-smacking dressing. It goes well with bitter salads and fish, and even makes a great sauce for roast beef or lamb, enhancing the flavours of the meat. Offers a good dose of healthy omega 3 fats too.

Serves about 4

4 tbsp extra-virgin olive oil

2 tsp rosemary leaves, very finely chopped

Juice of 1 lemon

5-6 salted anchovies from a jar, finely chopped

1 tsp wholegrain mustard

1 tsp honey

• DAIRY-FREE

• GLUTEN-FREE

• GOOD FOR PHASE 1

Whisk together the olive oil, rosemary, lemon juice and anchovies. Stir in the mustard and honey and season with freshly ground black pepper. Store it in the fridge for up to a week.

Tip: as the anchovies are salty, there is no need to add salt to this dressing.

130 CALORIES

Lime Dressing

Citrus-scented and full of flavour, this dressing is great with any kind of fish.

Serves about 4

4 tbsp olive oil

2 tbsp lime juice

½ tsp wholegrain mustard

1 tsp fresh mint or 1 tbsp fresh coriander, finely chopped

• DAIRY-FREE

• GLUTEN-FREE

• GOOD FOR PHASE 1

Mix all the ingredients together in a jar and store it in the fridge.

120 CALORIES

Salsa Verde with Seaweed

A super-healthy dressing, which is wonderful to pour over fish or to add a bit of zing to vegetables or salads.

Serves about 4

3 anchovy fillets in oil, from a jar

3-4 tbsp soft-leaf herbs, such as parsley, basil, oregano and mint, chopped

1½ tbsp live apple cider vinegar

5 tbsp extra-virgin olive oil

1 small garlic clove, crushed

1 tsp capers, rinsed

1 nori seaweed sheet, chopped (optional)

• DAIRY-FREE
• GLUTEN-FREE
• GOOD FOR PHASE 1

Blitz all the ingredients together in a blender. Store the dressing in the fridge for up to a week.

Tip: don't use too much mint, as it can overwhelm the other flavours. But a hint tastes great!

150 CALORIES

Live Apple Cider Vinegar Dressing

This classic dressing is sweet and tangy, and provides a great boost for your microbiome. Ideal to add to any bitter leaf salad.

Serves about 6

100ml extra-virgin olive oil

2 tbsp live apple cider vinegar

½ tbsp lemon juice

1 tsp maple syrup or honey

• DAIRY-FREE
• GLUTEN-FREE
• GOOD FOR PHASE 1

Mix all the ingredients together in a jar and store it in the fridge.

140 CALORIES

Kefir and Live Cultured Buttermilk Dressings

Kefir is one of the best sources of probiotics you will find, as it contains complex, acid-tolerant bacteria that are able to make it down to your microbiome in beneficial numbers. And, as ever, homemade is the best (page 190). Use it in place of a yoghurt-based dressing. Buttermilk is the name given to a variety of traditional fermented milks found in the Middle East, Eastern Europe, Scandinavia, India and other parts of Asia. In Britain, it was originally made from the liquid left over after churning butter from cream. These fermented milk dressings are all gluten-free, and are wonderfully enriching to almost any dish.

Lemony Buttermilk

A great dressing for salads and slaws. It delivers a double hit of different gut-friendly microbes from both the buttermilk and the preserved lemons.

Serves about 4

140ml live cultured
  buttermilk (or kefir)
½ tsp English mustard
3 tbsp extra-virgin olive oil
½ tsp maple syrup
  (optional)
½ tbsp Preserved Lemons
  (page 184), finely
  diced (or juice and grated
  zest of ½ small lemon)
½ tsp xanthum gum
  (optional thickener)

Whisk the buttermilk and mustard together in a bowl and gradually add the olive oil, followed by the maple syrup if using, and the preserved lemon. Season well with sea salt and freshly ground black pepper.

70 CALORIES

Kefir Mustard

Serves about 4
100ml kefir (or live cultured
   buttermilk)
2 tbsp extra-virgin olive oil
2 tsp wholegrain mustard
½ tsp xanthum gum
   (optional thickener)

Whisk all the ingredients together in a jar, season to taste and store it in the fridge for up to a week.

80 CALORIES

Creamy Pesto Kefir

A gutsy green dressing – and a great way to use up leftover Pistachio Pesto (page 99) and homemade Kefir Milk (page 190).

Serves about 4
125ml kefir
   (or live cultured
   buttermilk)
2 tbsp Pistachio Pesto 1
tbsp Parmesan, grated
½ tsp xanthum gum
   (optional thickener)

Whisk all the ingredients together in a jar, season to taste and store it in the fridge for up to a week.

90 CALORIES

Turmeric Buttermilk

Serves about 4
100ml live cultured
   buttermilk (or kefir)
Juice of ½ large lemon
2 tbsp olive oil
1 tsp English mustard
1 tsp ground turmeric
½ tsp xanthum gum
   (optional thickener)

Whisk together the buttermilk and lemon juice. Gradually whisk in the olive oil, mustard and turmeric. Season to taste with sea salt and plenty of black pepper.

• ALL GLUTEN-FREE

70 CALORIES

Flavourings

The two mantras of the Clever Guts Diet are eat more veg and eat a greater variety of ingredients overall. These flavourings will have you longing for a plate of mixed veg to add them to. The butters can be stored in the freezer, ready to dollop on when you are ready. And the Nut Butter (page 123) will add protein and nutrients to all sorts of dishes, sweet and savoury.

Dry Coconut Sambal

This Sri Lankan coconut mixture is full of good things, including turmeric, and can be guaranteed to spice things up. It's also a tasty way to enjoy some gut-friendly seaweed, though this is an optional addition.

Serves 6

2 tsp ground turmeric (or fresh grated)

3 tbsp desiccated coconut

1 tbsp nam pla (Thai fish sauce)

1 tbsp tamari (or soy) sauce

Juice of ½ lime

½-1 nori seaweed sheet, finely chopped (optional)

½ tsp chilli flakes (optional)

• DAIRY-FREE

• GLUTEN-FREE

• GOOD FOR PHASE 1

Mix everything together. You can enhance the flavours by grinding the mixture with a pestle and mortar. Store it in the fridge in a resealable jar.

5 Flavoured Butters

Allow the butter to soften at room temperature before beating it with the other ingredients. Chill it in the fridge for 10 minutes and then roll it into sausage shapes between sheets of baking paper to be sliced into discs and stored in the fridge (up to 1 month) or frozen.

Each makes 12 portions

Garlic and Parsley Butter

250g butter
3 garlic cloves, crushed
4 tbsp fresh parsley,
    finely chopped

Tip: add 1 tsp dried or 2 tsp fresh tarragon and use it to baste or stuff a chicken.

Herb Butter

250g butter
3 tbsp fresh herbs, such as
    thyme, oregano or
    rosemary, finely chopped

Tip: you could also mash in ½ tbsp diced anchovies to jazz up cooked vegetables.

Wholegrain Mustard Butter

250g butter
1 tbsp wholegrain mustard
1 garlic clove, crushed
1 tbsp capers, drained,
    rinsed, dried and
    chopped

Tip: dollop this butter on to grilled or baked fish, or steaming-hot green vegetables.

Lemon and Pepper Butter

250g butter
Grated zest of 2 lemons
1 tbsp fresh parsley,
    chopped
2 tsp freshly ground pink
    and black pepper

Tip: delicious on fish or freshly steamed asparagus.

Blue Cheese Butter

250g butter
100g blue cheese, such as
    Stilton or Roquefort

Tip: top a cooked burger with this butter, and ditch the starchy bun.

•ALL GLUTEN-FREE

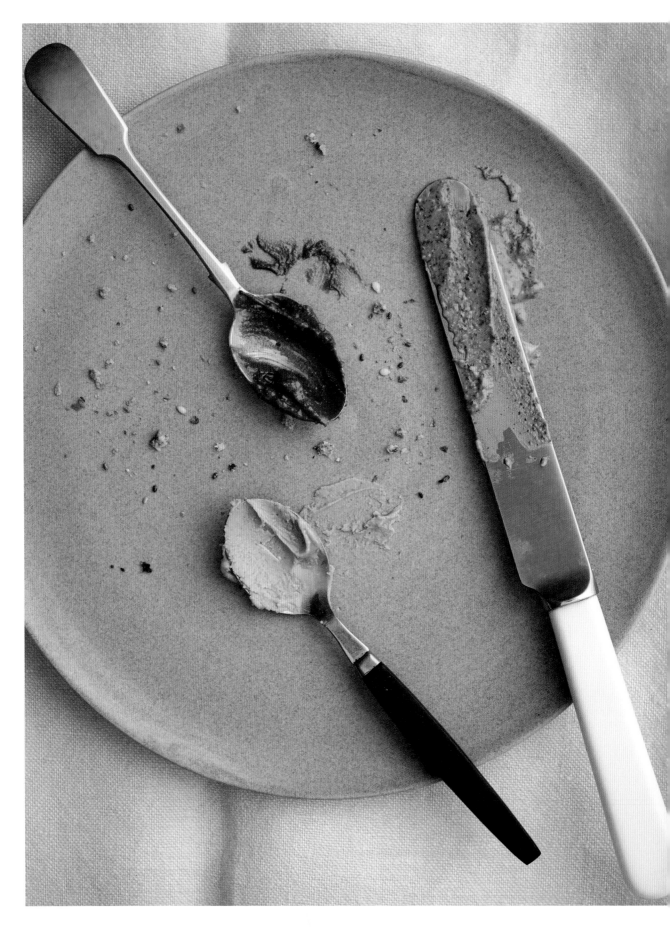

Nut Butter

There are myriad uses for nut butter, as well as eating it straight from the jar, as Michael sometimes does. Try spreading it on blinis or toast, baking with it, using it to thicken savoury sauces or dips, or adding it to smoothies for extra protein. It's also delicious stirred into dressings.

Makes 1 small jar,
16 portions (each one
= approx 1 tbsp)

250g nuts, such as
   almonds, unsalted
   peanuts, macadamias or
   cashews

1 tbsp coconut oil

• DAIRY-FREE
• GLUTEN-FREE
• GOOD FOR PHASE 1

1. Whizz the nuts to a fine powder in a blender or food processor. This can take 5-10 minutes, depending on the nuts used.

2. Then add the coconut oil to loosen the mixture and whizz it again for up to 5 minutes until it turns into a creamy paste.

3. Store it in a resealable jar in the fridge for up to 4 weeks.

Tip: using whole nuts, such as almonds with skin on rather than blanched, means all that fabulous fibre makes its way down the gut to boost your biome.

110 CALORIES

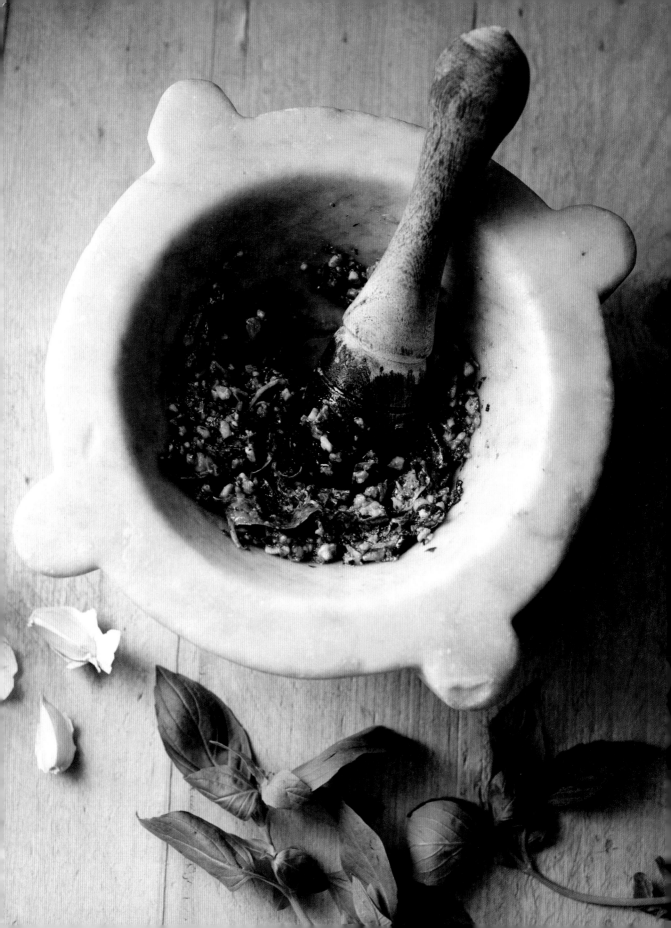

MAIN DISHES

It's best to eat most of your food earlier
in the day if you can – evidence shows
that you are less likely to store it as fat.
Try and do as the Mediterraneans do
and have your main meal at lunchtime,
followed by a light meal or snack
in the evening.

Poultry

Chicken and turkey are rich in protein. And birds raised with space to roam tend to contain more of the good stuff. Buy the best quality you can.

Baked Coconut Chicken Curry

This aromatic curry is bursting with goodness. Baking it in the oven gives the chicken a delicious crispy skin.

Serves 4

Juice and zest of 2 limes

2 garlic cloves, diced

1 tsp ground turmeric

2 tsp medium curry powder

½ tsp cayenne pepper
   or chilli flakes to taste
   (optional)

4 large chicken thighs, bone
   in and skin on

3 tbsp coconut oil, olive oil
   or ghee

1 onion, diced

2 medium red peppers,
   deseeded and sliced
   lengthways

1 tbsp Thai fish sauce
   (or soy sauce)

200ml coconut milk

2 bay leaves

Generous handful of fresh
coriander, roughly chopped

• DAIRY-FREE

• GLUTEN-FREE

• GOOD FOR PHASE 1

1. In a medium-sized bowl, mix together the lime juice and zest, garlic, turmeric, curry powder and cayenne pepper, if using. Coat the chicken pieces in the mixture and season them generously with salt and freshly ground black pepper. Leave them to marinate for at least 1 hour or overnight in the fridge.

2. Preheat the oven to 180°C/160°C fan/gas mark 4. Place a large casserole over a medium heat, add the oil and fry the diced onions and marinated chicken pieces, skin side down, for 4-5 minutes or until the chicken skin is just turning golden brown. Turn them over and seal the other side for 1-2 minutes.

3. Reduce the heat, add the red peppers and any remaining marinade, along with the fish sauce, coconut milk and bay leaves, and bring everything to a simmer.

4. Place the casserole in the middle of the oven for 25 minutes, basting the chicken occasionally, until it is cooked through. Remove it from the oven and stir in the coriander. Serve with a dollop of Greek-style yoghurt (add 75 cals), 2 tbsp brown rice (add 100 cals) and steamed green veg (add 20 cals).

880 CALORIES

Easy Chicken Tagine with Preserved Lemons

The North African equivalent of comfort food. Slow-cooked meat and vegetables are easier to digest, enabling you to absorb more nutrients, and leaving your digestive system with less work to do.

Serves 4

3 tbsp olive oil

1 large onion, diced

4 skinless and boneless chicken thighs (about 600g)

2 garlic cloves, finely chopped

4-5cm root ginger, peeled and diced

2 tsp ground cinnamon

2 tsp ground turmeric

2 tsp paprika

400ml chicken stock

1 large red pepper, deseeded and sliced

1 heaped tbsp Preserved Lemons, diced (page 184), or ½ lemon (removed before serving)

80g dried apricots, halved

Generous handful of fresh coriander, chopped

• DAIRY-FREE
• GLUTEN-FREE
• GOOD FOR PHASE 1

1. Preheat the oven to 150°C/130°C fan/gas mark 2. Heat the olive oil in a medium-sized casserole and sauté the onion for 2-3 minutes. Add the chicken pieces and brown them all over.

2. Stir in the garlic, ginger and spices and cook for a couple more minutes. Pour over the stock, then add the pepper, preserved lemon and apricots. Cover the casserole and place it in the oven for 1-1½ hours, stirring occasionally.

3. Stir the coriander into the chicken tagine just before serving. Serve it with 1 tbsp Greek-style yoghurt (add 75 cals) and 2 tbsp brown rice (add 100 cals) or 2 tbsp quinoa (add 120 cals).

Tip: ideally, use rice or quinoa that has been in the fridge or freezer for over 12 hours so that some of the starch is converted to more gut-friendly resistant starch.

470 CALORIES

Veira's Coriander Chicken with Yoghurt and Fennel

A light, tangy dish adapted from a recipe my mother learnt while living in Malaysia.

Serves 4

2 garlic cloves, diced

3cm root ginger, grated or finely chopped

Zest and juice of 2 limes

4 good-sized chicken thighs (approx 600g), bone in and skin on

3 tbsp coconut or rapeseed oil

1 large onion, diced

Seeds from 6 cardamom pods

2 fennel bulbs, trimmed and quartered lengthwise

2 celery stalks, diced

1 tsp cornflour

Large bunch of fresh coriander, chopped

300g full-fat live Greek-style yoghurt (or non-dairy equivalent)

1 green chilli, deseeded and diced

• DAIRY-FREE OPTION
• GLUTEN-FREE
• GOOD FOR PHASE 1

1. In a non-metallic bowl, mix together the garlic, ginger and the juice of 1 lime and the zest of both with some seasoning. Marinate the chicken in the mixture in the fridge for at least 1 hour, or ideally overnight.

2. Preheat the oven to 180°C/160°C fan/gas mark 4. Heat the coconut oil in a large frying pan and fry the chicken and onion on a medium heat for 8-10 minutes, turning occasionally, until they are lightly golden. Add the cardamom seeds for the last 2 minutes of cooking, then spoon the contents into a large baking dish. Tuck the fennel and celery between the chicken pieces.

3. Pour the rest of the lime juice and any remaining marinade into the frying pan to deglaze it. Stir in the cornflour and most of the coriander, followed by the yoghurt. Mix everything together thoroughly, scraping the pan to incorporate all the chicken juices, then pour it over the chicken in the baking dish.

4. Cover the dish with a lid or foil and transfer it to the oven. After 15 minutes, remove the cover and cook for a further 15-20 minutes, or until the chicken is slightly browned. Before serving, scatter some green chilli and the remaining coriander on top.

5. This goes well with Cauliflower Rice with Coriander (page 174) and stir-fried greens (add 40 cals). For an extra yoghurt kick, mix 100g Greek-style yoghurt with 1 tbsp coriander and 1 tbsp lime juice and dollop it on top.

650 CALORIES

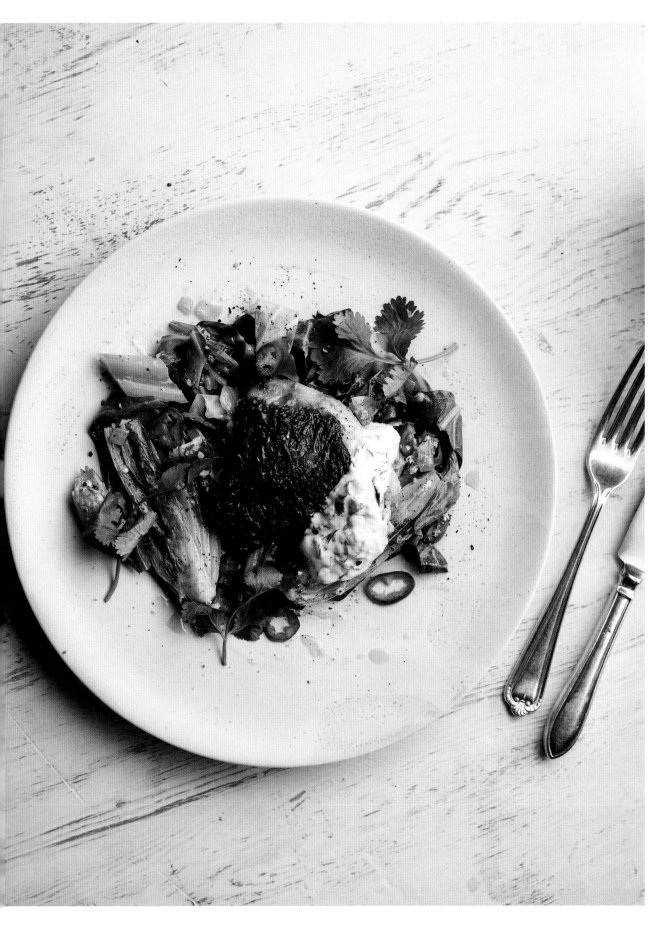

Lazy Lemon and Lime Baked Chicken

We have cooked many versions of this dish over the years and love the way the flavours are lifted by the preserved lemon. It is easy to preserve your own and they taste so much better than the stuff you buy in the shops.

Serves 4

Juice of 2 limes

2 garlic cloves, crushed

1½ tsp thyme leaves

1 tsp chilli flakes

4 boneless chicken thighs, skin on

3 tbsp olive oil

125g mushrooms, sliced

2 medium onions, sliced

1 Preserved Lemon, cut into wedges (see page 184)

175g mixed red and white quinoa or gluten-free bulgar wheat and quinoa

400ml hot chicken stock

• DAIRY-FREE

• GLUTEN-FREE

• GOOD FOR PHASE 1

1. Make a marinade with the lime juice, garlic, thyme and chilli flakes. Pour it over the chicken in a non-metallic bowl and leave it to stand for 1 hour, or up to 12 hours in the fridge.

2. Heat the oil in a frying pan and brown the chicken all over. Meanwhile, spread the mushrooms, onions and preserved lemon wedges over the bottom of a flameproof casserole or large saucepan. Sprinkle over the quinoa, then place the browned chicken on top.

3. Use half the stock to deglaze the frying pan and pour it over the chicken. Then add the remaining stock.

4. Let it simmer gently for 35-40 minutes, checking from time to time that the quinoa has not absorbed all the stock, and top up with a little water if necessary. Serve it with a vegetable of your choice, such as griddled courgette slices or steamed cavolo nero leaves (add 20 cals).

560 CALORIES

Turkey and Mushroom Bolognese

Two great base ingredients here: turkey, which offers a nice alternative to beef, cooks more quickly and makes a really tasty Bolognese, and mushrooms, which are incredibly low in carbohydrates and full of gut-friendly fibre, with a texture that is almost like meat. We love them.

Serves 4

4 tbsp olive oil

1 large red onion, diced

1 garlic clove, crushed

400g chestnut mushrooms, thinly sliced

300g turkey mince

2 x 400g cans chopped tomatoes

2 medium carrots, grated

2 bay leaves

1 tsp dried mixed herbs

600g spiralised butternut squash or courgetti to serve

• DAIRY-FREE OPTION

• GLUTEN-FREE

• GOOD FOR PHASE 1

1. Heat the oil in a pan and sauté the onion for 5-6 minutes. Add the garlic and mushrooms and cook for a further 3-4 minutes, stirring occasionally.

2. Stir in the turkey mince and cook for 4-5 minutes, then add the tomatoes, carrots, bay leaves and herbs. Season with salt and pepper, and leave it to simmer for 18-20 minutes.

3. Meanwhile, steam the spiralised butternut squash or courgetti. Divide it between 4 warmed plates and top with the Bolognese to serve.

510 CALORIES

Fish

One of the healthiest foods on the planet, fish is loaded with important nutrients which most of us don't get enough of. Try and eat it at least twice a week, choosing responsibly sourced varieties where possible.

Baked Salmon with Seaweed Pesto

A classic recipe for baked salmon, enhanced by the delicious umami flavours of gut-friendly, nutrient-packed seaweed.

Serves 4

3 red peppers, cut into
   large pieces
2 medium courgettes, sliced
2 red onions, cut into
   wedges
2 tbsp olive oil
4 tbsp pesto (make your
   own, page 90)
1½ nori seaweed sheets,
   chopped
4 x 150g salmon fillets

•DAIRY-FREE
•GLUTEN-FREE
•GOOD FOR PHASE 1

1. Preheat the oven to 180°C/160°C fan/gas mark 4. Place the peppers, courgettes and red onions in a large roasting tin, toss them in the olive oil and bake them for 12-15 minutes.

2. Meanwhile, stir the nori into the pesto and spread the mixture over the salmon fillets.

3. Place the salmon on top of the roasted vegetables and cover the tin with foil. Transfer it to the oven for 15 minutes, removing the foil for the last 5 minutes (don't overcook the salmon as it will dry out).

4. Serve the fish with a leafy green salad. It works well drizzled with Creamy Pesto Kefir Dressing (page 119).

540 CALORIES

Mackerel Fillets with Spiced Coconut

Mackerel is great value, and provides more omega 3 oil than almost any other fish. The tangy flavours in this crispy sambal topping really pep it up.

Serves 2
2 good-sized mackerel fillets
1 egg white
2 tbsp Dry Coconut Sambal
  (page 120)
Juice of ½ lime

•DAIRY-FREE

•GLUTEN-FREE

•GOOD FOR PHASE 1

1. Preheat the oven to 160°C/140°C fan/gas mark 3. Place the mackerel fillets skin side down in a lightly greased baking dish.

2. In a small bowl, lightly whisk the egg white, then stir in the sambal with some seasoning. Spread the mixture over the mackerel fillets and leave them to marinate in the fridge for up to 2 hours, if possible.

3. Bake the fillets in the oven for 12-15 minutes, or until the surface becomes crisp. Serve them with cooked quinoa (for 2 tbsp add 120 cals) and Scorched Purple Radicchio (page 160).

510 CALORIES

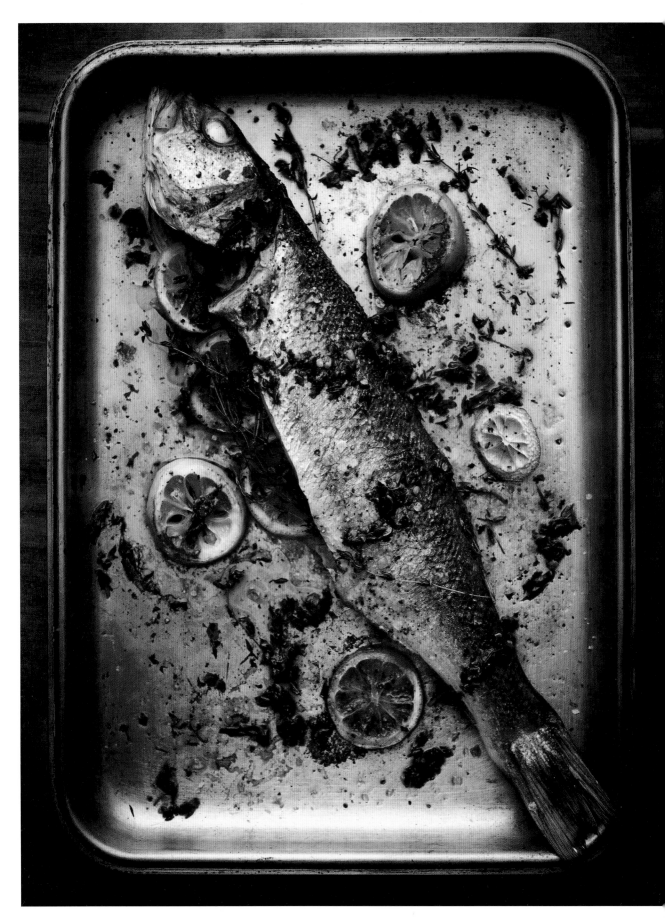

Sea Bass with Seaweed Salsa Verde

Crisp, succulent and full of flavours of the sea. A delicious way to top up your omega 3 and treat your microbiome to some seaweed.

Serves 2

1 tbsp olive or rapeseed oil

2 sea bass fillets

Salsa Verde with Seaweed
  (page 117)

•DAIRY-FREE

•GLUTEN-FREE

•GOOD FOR PHASE 1

1. Place a frying pan over a medium heat, add the oil and fry the sea bass fillets skin side up for 4-5 minutes.

2. Turn the fillets over, then drizzle them with half of the Seaweed Salsa Verde. Cook them for a further 3-4 minutes before transferring them to a plate and pouring over the rest of the salsa.

3. Serve with 3-4 small boiled potatoes (ideally reheated so they contain more resistant starch; add 40 cals) and Pea and Edamame Mash (page 162).

Tip: if using a whole fish, stuff some seaweed salsa verde into the cavity for extra flavour.

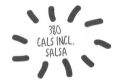

380 CALS INCL. SALSA

Sweet Potato, Kale and Cod Fishcakes

These Moroccan-flavoured fishcakes can also be made with other fish, such as salmon or trout. The sweet potatoes help bind them and are easy on the gut. They are delicious served with a crunchy green salad, or Green Beans and Edamame with Anchovies (page 87), or even for breakfast, topped with a poached egg.

Serves 4

700g sweet potatoes,
  peeled and chopped
30g kale, shredded
3 spring onions, finely
  chopped
1 tsp harissa paste
1 egg, beaten
260g cod fillet
3 tbsp buckwheat flour
2 tbsp olive oil

• DAIRY-FREE
• GLUTEN-FREE
• GOOD FOR PHASE 1

1. Steam the sweet potatoes for 6 minutes, then add the kale and steam for another 6-8 minutes, or until the potatoes are tender. Transfer the veg to a bowl and lightly mash them with a fork or potato masher. Add the spring onions, harissa and egg and season well.

2. Meanwhile, place the cod in a pan and cover it with water. Bring it to a simmer and cook it for 4-5 minutes, until the flesh flakes away from the skin easily. Add the flaked fish to the veg, stirring well with a fork to mix all the ingredients together. With wet hands, divide the mixture into 8 fishcakes. Dust them with a little flour and chill them in the fridge for 20 minutes.

3. Heat the oil in a frying pan and fry the fishcakes for 3-4 minutes on each side, or until they are golden. You might serve them with Creamy Nutmeg Spinach (page 160) and Puy Lentils with Balsamic Vinegar (page 169).

340 CALORIES

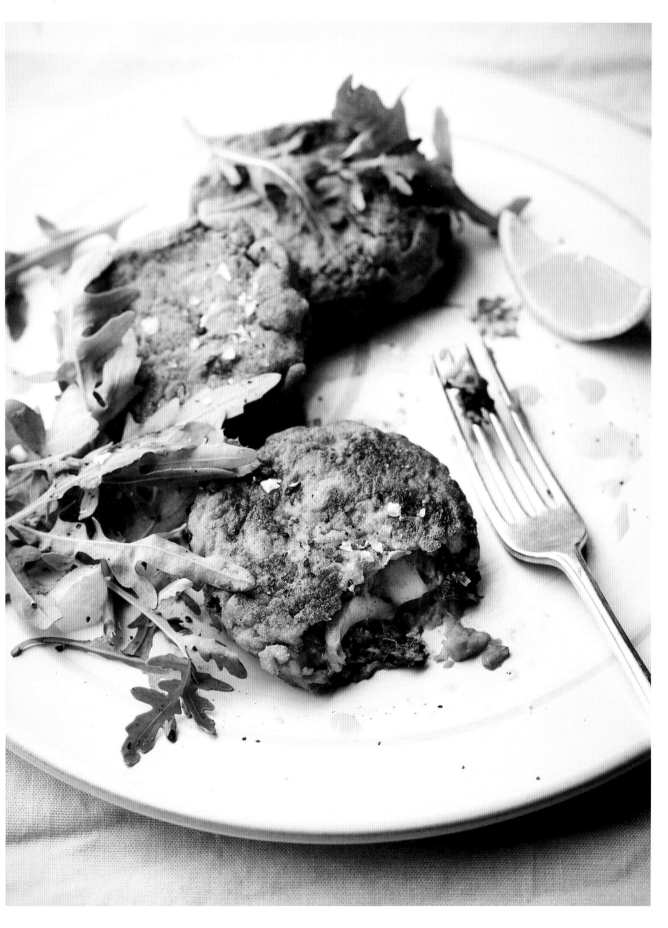

Seafood

You will have noticed that nearly all of our fish and seafood recipes contain seaweed. It is not key to the dishes, so it can be reduced or left out altogether if you prefer. But sprinkle it on liberally if you can. It adds a wonderful salty, seafoody taste and your microbiome thrives on it...

Prawns with Pasta and Seaweed

We love prawns and they work brilliantly in this easy Mediterranean-style pasta dish. And here's that seaweed again.

Serves 2

250g wholewheat (or gluten-free) pasta
4 tbsp olive oil
2 celery stalks, diced
½ fennel bulb, sliced
4 spring onions, trimmed and sliced
2 garlic cloves, diced
50g anchovies from a jar, drained and chopped
½ tsp dried thyme
350g prawns (fresh or frozen, defrosted)
185g frozen spinach, defrosted
2 nori seaweed sheets, finely chopped
Juice of 1 lemon
¼ tsp Tabasco sauce to taste

•DAIRY-FREE
•GLUTEN-FREE OPTION
•GOOD FOR PHASE 1

1. Cook the pasta according to the pack instructions.

2. Meanwhile, in a large deep frying pan, heat the olive oil and sauté the celery, fennel, spring onions and garlic for 4-5 minutes, until they're soft but not brown. Add the anchovies and thyme and cook for a further couple of minutes.

3. Add the prawns, spinach and nori, along with the lemon juice, Tabasco, and some salt and black pepper.

4. Add the drained pasta to the pan, tossing it well to coat it with the sauce. Serve it with a multicoloured salad (add 20 cals).

880 CALORIES

Seafood with Seaweed Risotto

We recommend eating lots of different kinds of seafood – and this risotto gives you the opportunity to do just that. You can buy frozen mixes containing mussels, squid and prawns in most supermarkets.

Serves 2

700ml vegetable stock

3 tbsp olive oil

1 small onion, diced

1 large garlic clove, chopped

225g brown rice

400g frozen mixed seafood, defrosted

100ml white wine

Juice of 1 lemon

2 tbsp fresh parsley, chopped

1½ nori seaweed sheets, chopped

2 tbsp Parmesan (or vegan Parmesan), grated

½ tsp chilli flakes (optional)

• DAIRY-FREE OPTION
• GLUTEN-FREE
• GOOD FOR PHASE 1

1. Bring the stock to a simmer in a saucepan.

2. Heat 2 tbsp of the olive oil in a another larger saucepan and sauté the onions and garlic for 3-4 minutes or until they start to soften. Add the rice and stir for a couple of minutes, before pouring over enough stock to cover it. Leave it to simmer, covered, stirring occasionally and topping up with stock as the rice absorbs it.

3. When the rice has been cooking for around 10 minutes, heat the remaining oil in a frying pan and stir-fry the seafood for 2-3 minutes, then spoon it into the risotto.

4. Deglaze the frying pan with the wine, then pour it into the risotto too. Continue to top up the risotto with stock for around 30 minutes, by which time the rice should be cooked al dente. Serve it with a bitter leaf salad (pages 54-56) or cooked greens (add 20 cals).

560 CALORIES

Prawns are high in protein, low in calories and a good source of vitamin D, vitamin B12, iron and selenium.

Thai Prawns with Coconut Milk and Seaweed

Simple to make and packed with health-boosting antioxidants.

Serves 2

140g green-pea pasta
  (or wholemeal pasta)
150g broccoli, broken into
  florets
3 tbsp coconut oil
½ red onion, sliced
2cm root ginger, grated
½ red chilli, deseeded and
    finely chopped (or ¼ tsp
    chilli flakes)
200ml coconut milk
Juice of 1 lime
½ tbsp Thai fish sauce
2 nori seaweed sheets,
    chopped
200g prawns (fresh or
    frozen, defrosted)
Generous handful of fresh
    coriander, chopped

• DAIRY-FREE
• GLUTEN-FREE
• GOOD FOR PHASE 1

1. Cook the pasta according to the pack instructions.

2. Steam the broccoli for 4-5 minutes and set it aside.

3. Heat the oil in a large frying pan and sauté the onion for 4-5 minutes. Add the ginger and chilli, cook for 1 minute and then pour in the coconut milk, lime juice, fish sauce, seaweed and prawns.

4. Bring the pan to a simmer, then add the broccoli and simmer for 2 minutes more before stirring in the pasta with the coriander. Serve immediately.

700 CALORIES

Squid Provençal

This makes a gorgeous, deep-red, herby stew. Squid is good value and an excellent source of protein.

Serves 2

3 tbsp olive oil

1 small onion, sliced

1 red pepper, deseeded and finely diced

2 garlic cloves, finely chopped

1 tsp thyme, fresh or dried

2 bay leaves

400g can chopped tomatoes

100ml white wine

½ tsp chilli flakes

300g prepared squid (defrosted frozen is fine)

Handful of fresh parsley or coriander, chopped, to serve

• DAIRY-FREE

• GLUTEN-FREE

• GOOD FOR PHASE 1

1. Heat the oil in a pan and sauté the onion, pepper and garlic for 3-4 minutes. Add the thyme and bay leaves, along with the tomatoes, wine and chilli flakes, and simmer for 10 minutes.

2. Turn the heat down as low as you can, add the squid and simmer very gently or place the pan in the oven, covered, at 100°C for about 50 minutes. Don't actually boil it as it will become rubbery.

3. To thicken the sauce, remove 1-2 cupfuls of it with a ladle and blitz it in a blender, then return it to the pan. Serve the stew with 2 tbsp brown rice (ideally cooled and reheated to increase resistant starch; add 100 cals) or quinoa (add 120 cals) and a multicoloured leafy salad (add 20 cals).

430 CALORIES

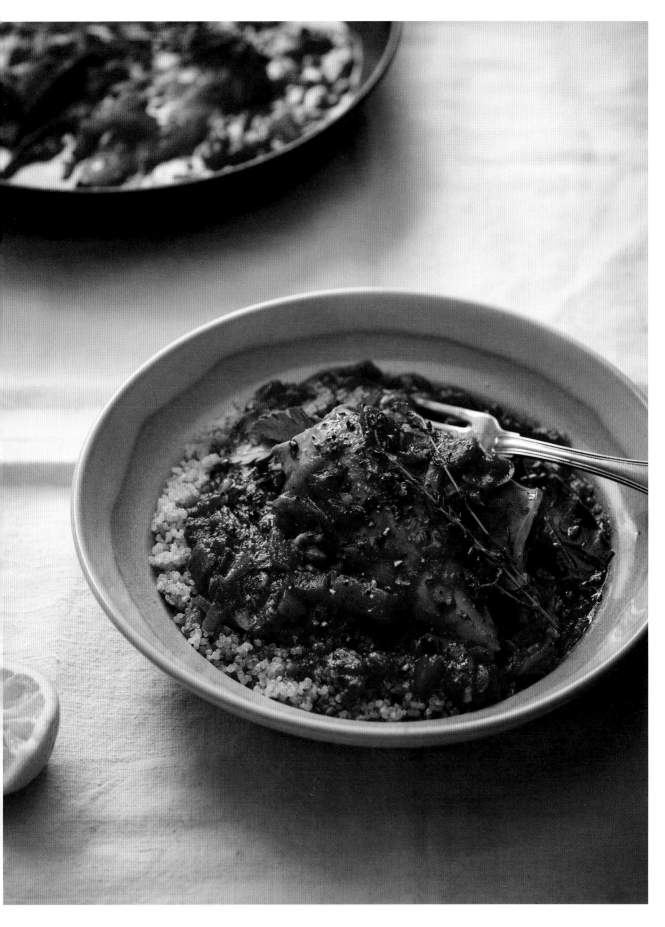

Vegetable Dishes

There are many quick vegetarian dishes elsewhere in this book. These recipes take a bit longer to prepare but are definitely worth the effort.

Marinated Tofu Stir-Fry with Noodles

Marinating and then baking tofu transforms it from something pale and rather bland into a flavoursome delicacy – so tasty you could nibble it on its own.

Serves 2

2 tbsp tamari sauce (or soy sauce)
1 garlic clove, crushed
2 tsp sesame oil (optional)
2cm root ginger, diced
225g silken tofu, drained and chopped into 1½cm pieces
100g soba noodles (or an alternative gluten-free noodle)
2 tbsp coconut oil
1 red pepper, deseeded and chopped
4 spring onions, sliced
125g tenderstem broccoli (ideally purple sprouting)
200ml vegetable stock
2 tbsp cashew nuts
150g bean sprouts
½ tsp chilli flakes (optional)

• DAIRY-FREE
• GLUTEN-FREE OPTION
• GOOD FOR PHASE 1

1. Preheat the oven to 160°C/140°C fan/gas mark 3 and line a baking tray with greaseproof paper.

2. In a medium-sized bowl, mix together the tamari, garlic, sesame oil and ginger. Gently toss the tofu in the marinade, and then spread it over the baking tray and season it with black pepper.

3. Bake the tofu for 30 minutes, turning it once halfway through cooking. It should be golden and crisp at the edges.

4. Cook the noodles in a pan of boiling water for 5 minutes or according to the pack instructions. Drain them and refresh them under cold running water.

5. Heat the coconut oil in a wok, and stir-fry the pepper, spring onions and broccoli for 2-3 minutes. Reduce the temperature and add 50ml of the stock. Continue to stir-fry for 3-4 minutes, before adding the cashews, tofu, bean sprouts and chilli flakes. Pour in the remaining stock with the noodles, bring it to a simmer and serve immediately.

410 CALORIES

Vegetable and Paneer Curry

An easy vegetarian curry with lots of flavour and not too spicy.

Serves 4

2 aubergines, diced

2 red peppers, deseeded
 and diced

½ small cauliflower, broken
 into florets

6 tbsp mild olive oil or
 rapeseed oil

2 onions, 1 diced and 1
 sliced into rings

2cm root ginger, peeled and
 chopped

2 garlic cloves, chopped

1 tsp mustard seeds

1 tsp ground turmeric

1 tsp cumin seeds

½-1 tsp chilli flakes

400g can chopped tomatoes

250ml vegetable stock

175g paneer or tofu, sliced

Handful of fresh coriander,
 chopped

• DAIRY-FREE OPTION

• GLUTEN-FREE

• GOOD FOR PHASE 1

1. Preheat the oven to 200°C/180°C fan/gas mark 6. Spread the aubergine, peppers and cauliflower in the base of a roasting tin. Drizzle with 2 tbsp of the olive oil and season with a pinch of salt. Bake the vegetables for 15-20 minutes or until they start to caramelise, turning them once.

2. Heat 2 tbsp of the oil in a frying pan and fry the onion rings, stirring frequently, until they're crisp and golden brown. Set them aside.

3. Heat the remaining oil in a medium-sized casserole and sauté the diced onions for 4-5 minutes before adding the ginger, garlic and spices. Cook for 2 more minutes.

4. Remove the vegetables from the oven and spoon them into the casserole, stirring to give them a good coating of the spice mixture. Pour in the chopped tomatoes and stock and bring to the boil. Simmer for 15-20 minutes. Stir in the paneer cheese (or tofu) for the last 5 minutes. Season to taste with salt and black pepper and stir in most of the coriander. Scatter the rest over the top, along with the fried onion rings.

5. Serve with Cauliflower and Coriander Rice (page 174) or 2 tbsp brown basmati rice (100 cals), 1 tbsp Greek-style yoghurt (75 cals) and Onion and Courgette Bhajis (page 162).

430 CALORIES

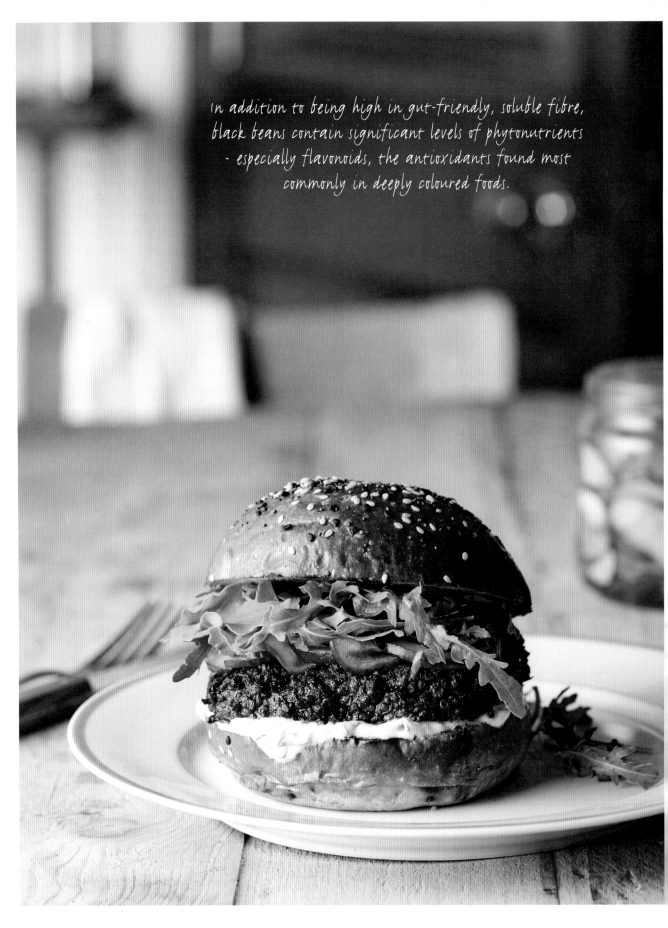

In addition to being high in gut-friendly, soluble fibre, black beans contain significant levels of phytonutrients - especially flavonoids, the antioxidants found most commonly in deeply coloured foods.

Black Bean Beet Burgers

These burgers look so like beef burgers they are in danger of putting off vegetarians. A seeded bun makes them a real treat.

Makes 4

150g beetroot, peeled
  and diced into ½cm pieces
1 small onion, finely diced
½ tsp ground cumin
1 tsp ground coriander
3 tbsp olive oil
400g can black beans
  (or kidney beans), drained
  but not rinsed
1 large garlic clove, crushed
½ tsp chilli flakes
Zest of 2 limes
1 medium egg, beaten
150g precooked quinoa
  (red, white or black)
40g vegan Parmesan, grated
2 tbsp fresh parsley,
chopped

•DAIRY-FREE
•GLUTEN-FREE
•GOOD FOR PHASE 1

1. Preheat the oven to 180°C/160°C fan/gas mark 4. Mix the beetroot and onion together in a medium-sized bowl with the cumin, coriander, 1 tbsp of the olive oil and some seasoning. Spoon the mixture into a roasting tin and bake it, covered, in the oven for 20-25 minutes, until the beetroot starts to soften.

2. Meanwhile, place the beans, garlic, chilli flakes and lime zest in the bowl used for the beetroot. Season with salt and black pepper and mash with a fork or a hand blender, leaving some texture.

3. When the beetroot is cooked, allow it to cool for 10 minutes before mixing it into the beans. Then add the egg, quinoa, Parmesan and parsley, and mix thoroughly. With wet hands, shape the mixture into 8 medium-sized burgers, and chill them in the fridge for 20 minutes.

4. Heat the remaining oil in a frying pan and cook the burgers on a medium heat for 5-6 minutes on each side. Serve them with a wholegrain bun (add 100 cals) or Wholemeal Flatbread (page 195), with Pickled Courgette or Red Cabbage Sauerkraut (see pages 188 and 185), or on a plate with 2 tbsp bulgar wheat (add 100 cals) or quinoa (add 120 cals) and a salad such as Bitter Leaves with Toasted Pine Nuts (page 56).

Note: if you have IBS eat beans in moderation and avoid during the first two weeks of Phase 1 as beans can exacerbate symptoms.

280 CALORIES EXCL THE BUN

Quorn and Parsnip Cottage Pie

Quorn is made from mycoprotein, a fungus grown in a fermentation process similar to that used in the production of yoghurt, and is an excellent source of protein, fibre and nutrients. For a non-vegetarian version, use minced turkey or pork instead.

Serves 4

300g parsnips, scrubbed
  and diced into 2cm cubes
300g celeriac, scrubbed and
  diced into 2cm cubes
5 tbsp olive oil
1 onion, diced
2 bay leaves
1 tsp ground cumin
1 tsp ground cinnamon
350g Quorn mince
150g butternut squash,
  peeled and diced
400g can chopped tomatoes
1 tbsp apple cider vinegar
1 vegetable stock cube
100g spinach, chopped
2 tbsp Parmesan (or vegan
  Parmesan), grated

• DAIRY-FREE OPTION
• GLUTEN-FREE
• GOOD FOR PHASE 1

1. Preheat the oven to 180°C/160°C fan/gas mark 4. Cook the parsnips and celeriac in a pan of simmering salted water for 15-18 minutes, or until they're soft.

2. Meanwhile, in a large casserole with a lid, heat 3 tbsp of the olive oil and sauté the onion for 5 minutes, adding the spices and herbs halfway through. Add the Quorn mince and cook for 5-7 minutes, stirring frequently. Then mix in the diced squash along with the chopped tomatoes, cider vinegar, 200ml water and the crumbled stock cube. Simmer gently for about 10 minutes with the lid on and then season with salt and pepper.

3. Drain the parsnip and celeriac, return them to the pan and mash them vigorously with 1 tbsp olive oil and 1 tbsp Parmesan. Place a layer of spinach on top of the Quorn mixture, followed by the mash. Scatter the rest of the Parmesan on top and drizzle over the remaining olive oil.

4. Place the dish in the middle of the oven for 25-30 minutes, or until the pie is golden brown on top. Serve it with steamed greens (add 20 cals).

410 CALORIES

Red Meat

Red meat is fine for you in modest amounts and is an excellent source of protein and iron. We are gradually moving towards having red meat only about twice a week. The upside of this is that we find we are enjoying our vegetables more, both incorporated into the dish and as sides. In many of these dishes the vegetables contribute vital taste, texture and flavours.

Prosciutto-Wrapped Pork Loin

The prosciutto and cream cheese wrapping keeps the pork moist and succulent, and the roasted fennel adds a delicious sweetness.

Serves 4

140g cream cheese
2 garlic cloves, finely
  chopped
2 tsp fresh oregano,
  chopped (or 1 tsp dried)
500g pork loin
5 slices of prosciutto crudo
  or serrano ham
2 fennel bulbs, trimmed
  and quartered
2 tbsp olive oil

• DAIRY-FREE OPTION
• GLUTEN-FREE
• GOOD FOR PHASE 1

1. Preheat the oven to 180°C/160°C fan/gas mark 4. Mix together the cream cheese, garlic and oregano with some salt and black pepper. Spread the mixture over the pork loin and then wrap the prosciutto around it, covering as much of it as possible.

2. Place the pork in a roasting tin with the fennel quarters, and drizzle with the olive oil. Bake it in the oven for 30-35 minutes, basting it occasionally. It is cooked when the juices run clear.

3. Serve it sliced, with 2 tbsp quinoa (add 120 cals) and a large helping of dark-green leaves, such as cavolo nero, Swiss chard or spring greens (add 20 cals). Or add some Aubergine Chips (page 175).

Tip: for a non-dairy version, you can substitute the cream cheese with hummus.

420 CALORIES

Beef and Orange Stew with Mushrooms

The best of comfort food. Slow-cooked and gentle on the gut. Lots of lovely mushrooms too!

Serves 2

3 tbsp olive oil

1 large white onion, diced

300g stewing steak, diced

3cm root ginger, diced

2 bay leaves

1 star anise (optional)

250ml passata

1 tbsp apple cider vinegar

2 tsp Dijon mustard

Zest and juice of 1 orange

3 large celery stalks, diced

100g carrots, diced

1 organic beef or vegetarian
   stock cube

200g mushrooms, sliced

• DAIRY-FREE

• GLUTEN-FREE

• GOOD FOR PHASE 1

1. Preheat the oven to 160°C/140°C fan/gas mark 3. Heat the olive oil in a large casserole and sauté the onion for 5 minutes before adding the meat. Brown it all over, then add the ginger, bay leaves, star anise, passata, vinegar, mustard, orange zest and juice and mix well.

2. Tip in the celery and carrots, then crumble in the stock cube with just enough water to cover everything. Stir gently, bring it to a simmer and then cover the casserole and place it in the oven for 2-2 ½ hours, adding the mushrooms after 1 hour.

3. Check from time to time and add more water if needed. Season to taste with salt and black pepper. Serve with greens, such as steamed cavolo nero, kale or broccoli (add 20 cals), and 3-4 small new potatoes (add 40 cals).

700 CALORIES

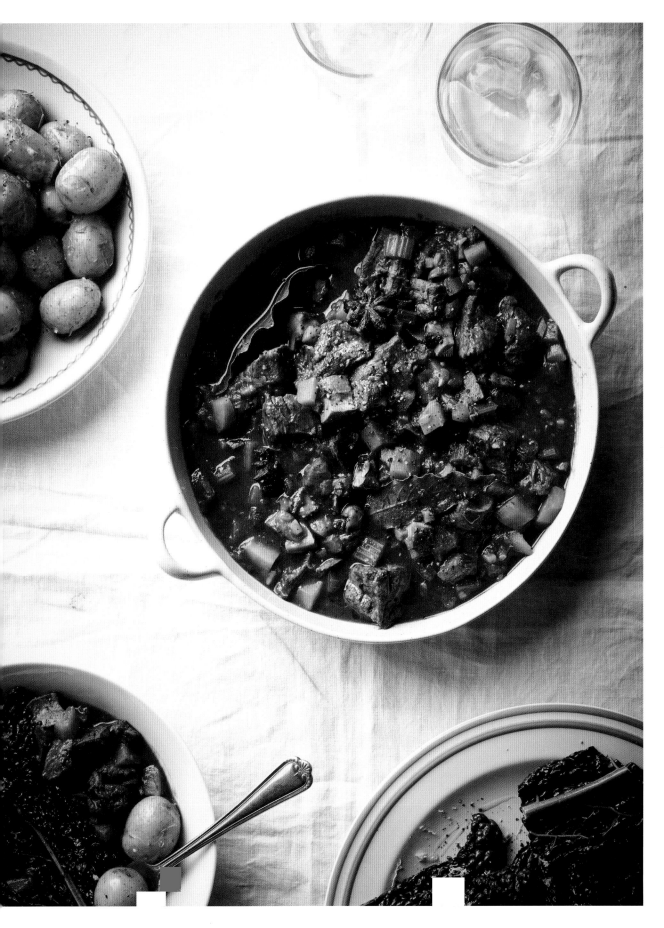

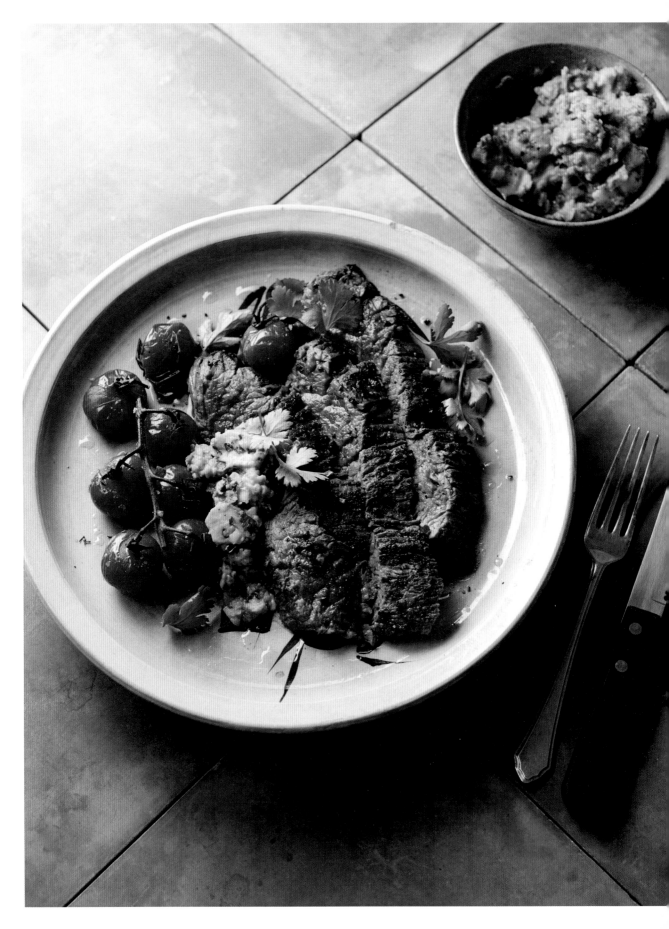

Steak with Guacamole and Blistered Tomatoes

Pounding the steak before you cook it, particularly if it's an economic cut or is fairly thick, will tenderise it and make it easier to digest. Marinating it, especially in an acidic element, such as lemon juice, will aid this process, and also enhance the flavour.

Serves 2

2 x 120g steaks, skirt
    or sirloin
1 tsp ground cumin
1 garlic clove, crushed
1 tbsp lemon juice
1 tbsp olive oil
1 avocado, diced
½ red onion, diced
½-1 tsp chilli flakes
1 tbsp fresh coriander
    or basil, chopped
1 tbsp lime juice
16 cherry tomatoes, halved

•DAIRY-FREE
•GLUTEN-FREE
•GOOD FOR PHASE 1

1. If using thick steaks, place them on a wooden chopping board and pound them with the rough side of a mallet. If you don't have a mallet you can use the end of a wooden rolling pin. Bash from the middle outwards. Don't pound the meat too hard or you will shred it.

2. In a bowl, mix together the cumin, garlic, lemon juice and olive oil. Place the steaks in a shallow dish and pour the mixture over them (turning them to make sure they are well covered). Leave them to marinate for 20 minutes.

3. Meanwhile, make the guacamole by mashing together the avocado, red onion, chilli flakes, coriander and lime juice. Season it with salt and pepper and set it aside.

4. Place a griddle or frying pan over a high heat. Cook the tomatoes, cut side up, for 3-4 minutes, until the skins are blistered. Remove them from the pan and add the steaks. Fry them for approximately 3 minutes on each side (for a medium steak).

5. Slice up the steaks, top them with the blistered tomatoes and serve the guacamole on the side.

470 CALORIES

Sausage and Mediterranean Veg Tray Bake

All cooked in one tray, and containing lots of fibre-rich vegetables.

Serves 2

4 good-quality free-range
  sausages (or gluten-free
  sausages)
1 red pepper, deseeded
  and sliced
1 yellow pepper, deseeded
  and sliced
1 medium red onion,
  cut into 8 wedges
3 tbsp olive oil
1 tsp dried thyme
  or oregano
1 medium courgette,
  cut into batons
100g cherry tomatoes
  on the vine
1½ tbsp balsamic vinegar
2 heaped tbsp cooked
  wholegrains (quinoa,
  bulgar wheat or pearl
  barley)

• DAIRY-FREE
• GLUTEN-FREE OPTION
• GOOD FOR PHASE 1

1. Preheat the oven to 180°C/160°C fan/gas mark 4. Place the sausages in a large roasting tray with the peppers and onion. Drizzle over the oil, and sprinkle the herbs, some Maldon sea salt and freshly ground black pepper on top.

2. Place the tray in the centre of the oven for 15 minutes, then stir in the courgette and tomatoes and drizzle over the balsamic vinegar. Return the tray to the oven for a further 10-15 minutes or until the sausages start to brown.

3. When they are cooked, stir in the wholegrains and serve.

510 CALORIES

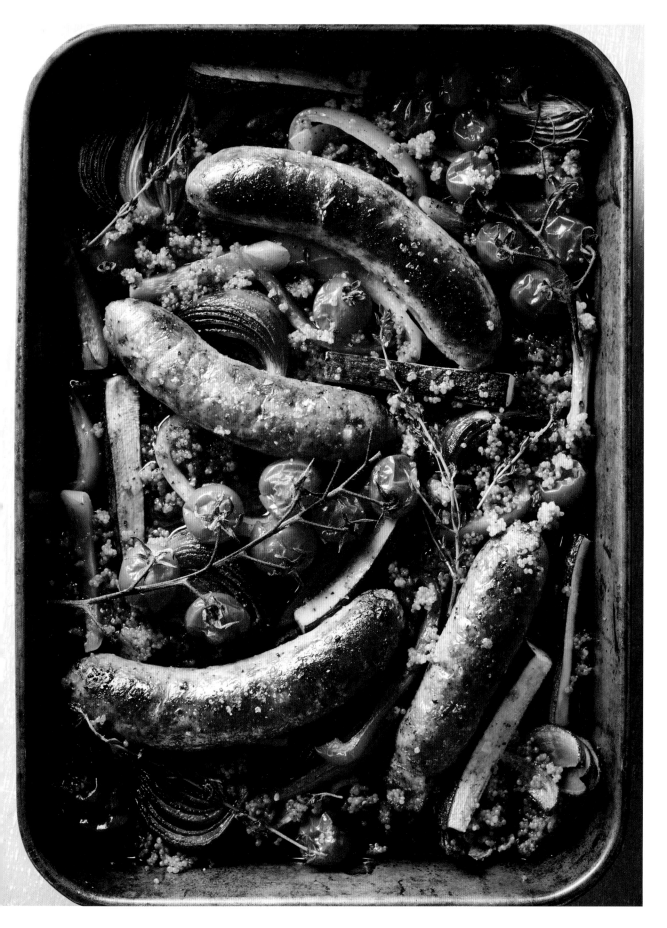

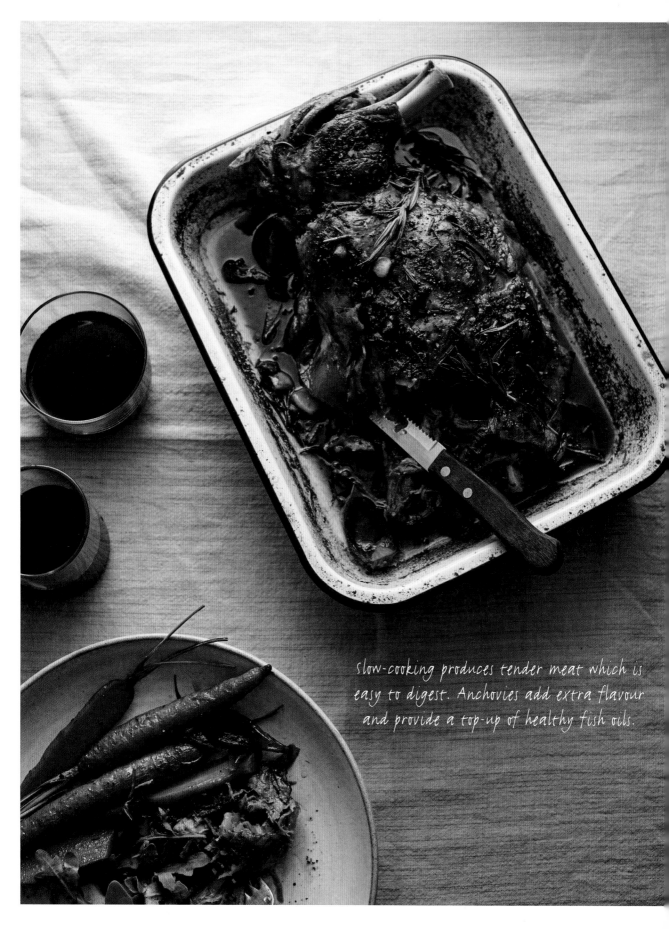

Slow-cooking produces tender meat which is easy to digest. Anchovies add extra flavour and provide a top-up of healthy fish oils.

Slow-Roast Shoulder of Lamb

The meat portions here are generous but not huge as this is not a particularly high-protein diet. Evidence suggests that, while we need a minimum daily amount of protein (around 45-60g) because we are unable to store it, eating significantly more is not necessarily better, unless you are doing a great deal of exercise.

Serves 8

3 garlic cloves, crushed

3 anchovies from a tin
  or jar, chopped

2 tbsp olive oil

Juice of 1 large lemon

3 sprigs of rosemary, leaves
  of 1 sprig, chopped

1¼kg shoulder of lamb

2 red onions, peeled
  and halved

1 glass of wine

• DAIRY-FREE

• GLUTEN-FREE

• GOOD FOR PHASE 1

1. Make a marinade by mixing together the garlic, anchovies, olive oil, lemon juice and chopped rosemary leaves. Slash the surface of the meat in several places and place it in a non-metallic dish. Rub in the marinade and leave the lamb to absorb the flavours and soften for 2-3 hours or overnight.

2. Take the lamb out of the fridge 30 minutes before cooking to bring it up to room temperature. Preheat the oven to 140°C/120°C fan/gas mark 1.

3. Place the onions in the base of a roasting tin with the marinated meat on top. Pour any remaining marinade over the meat and tuck the 2 rosemary sprigs underneath. Pour the wine into the tray, along with 100ml water. Cover the tray with a foil tent.

4. Roast the lamb for 4 hours, basting it occasionally. Top up with water as needed if the juices start to dry out. Remove the foil for the last 20-30 minutes of cooking time.

5. Serve the lamb with Cauliflower Baked with Lemon and Almonds (page 95), Roasted Purple Carrots (page 171) and greens of your choice (add 20 cals). There should be plenty of juices in the pan for gravy.

430 CALORIES

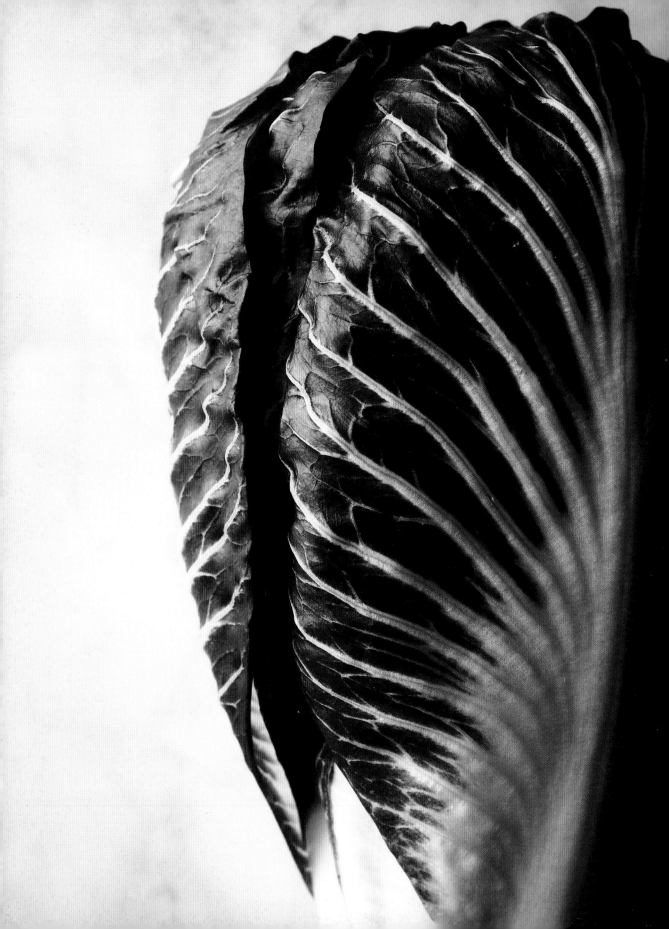

CLEVER VEG

Eating more veg is one
of the best ways of increasing the
diversity of your gut microbes,
and the greater the variety you
eat the better. Whatever you are
cooking, consider adding one of
these dishes on the side...

Creamy Nutmeg Spinach

A great way to jazz up spinach.

Serves 2

1 large knob of butter
  (or 1 tbsp light olive oil)
½ small onion, finely diced
1 garlic clove, crushed
½ tsp grated nutmeg
200g fresh spinach,
  tough stalks removed (or
  defrosted frozen spinach)
50g crème fraîche
  (or soya cream)
30g Parmesan (or vegan
  Parmesan), grated

• DAIRY-FREE OPTION
• GLUTEN-FREE
• GOOD FOR PHASE 1

1. Heat the oil in a frying pan or wok. Sauté the onion gently on a medium heat for 4-5 minutes, then add the garlic and nutmeg and cook for another 2 minutes.

2. Tip in the spinach and cook it, stirring occasionally, until it starts to wilt.

3. Add the crème fraîche and Parmesan and let it simmer for a couple of minutes. Serve it piping hot.

Note: can be made with either fresh or frozen and defrosted spinach.

240 CALORIES

Scorched Purple Radicchio

Charring the radicchio adds a wonderful caramelised, lightly smoked flavour to the leaves. The more bitter the leaves, the better they tend to be for both you and your microbiome.

Serves 2

½ radicchio, cut in half
Squeeze of lemon juice

• DAIRY-FREE
• GLUTEN-FREE
• GOOD FOR PHASE 1

1. Place the radicchio on a baking tray under a hot grill, cut side up, and season with salt and pepper. Grill it until the edges are starting to char, around 3 minutes.

2. Squeeze some lemon on top before serving.

Tip: the radicchio can also be cooked on a griddle or over a barbecue for enhanced smokiness.

10 CALORIES

Quick Garlic-Fried Greens

Do as the Mediterraneans do. Simple.

Serves 2

150g dark leaf greens, such
as mature spinach, spring
greens, cavolo nero, Swiss
chard or kale, chopped
and tough stalks removed

2 tbsp olive oil

1 garlic clove, finely
chopped

Grated zest of ½ lemon,
plus a small squeeze of
juice

20g Parmesan or pecorino
cheese (or vegan
Parmesan), grated

• DAIRY-FREE OPTION
• GLUTEN-FREE
• GOOD FOR PHASE 1

1. Steam or boil the greens until they are just starting
to soften, then drain them.

2. Heat the olive oil in a frying pan and add the garlic,
followed by the greens.

3. Sprinkle the lemon zest and Parmesan on top and
cook for a couple of minutes on a medium heat.
Season with freshly ground black pepper and a
squeeze of lemon.

Note: for most people, the 'scratchy', tough fibre in the stalks of
cabbage or kale, or the stringy bits in beans, is well tolerated,
particularly if chewed properly. But those with IBS may need to
reduce the amount they eat of it and go easy with pulses and
lentils, too, as these can exacerbate bloating and cramps. (For
more on FODMAPS in IBS see page 24).

290 CALORIES

Pea and Edamame Mash

Peas and edamame beans provide fibre, protein and other vital nutrients.

Serves 2
100g frozen edamame
100g frozen petit pois
2 tbsp full-fat fromage
   frais (or soya cream)
2-3 mint leaves, chopped
Juice of 1 lime

• DAIRY-FREE OPTION
• GLUTEN-FREE
• GOOD FOR PHASE 1

1. Bring a pan of salted water to the boil, and cook the edamame for 2-3 minutes before adding the frozen peas. Cook for a further 5 minutes, then drain them and transfer them to a bowl. Mix in the fromage frais, mint and lime juice. Season with salt and black pepper.

2. Using a potato masher, roughly mash most of the peas and beans, leaving some whole, until you have the consistency you like. For a smoother consistency, use a hand blender.

Note: if you have IBS, you might want to reduce your portion size.

150 CALORIES

Onion and Courgette Bhajis

These bhajis have been a huge hit in our household. Mixing turmeric with black pepper boosts its anti-inflammatory effect.

Serves 4
60g gram (chickpea)
   flour
½ tsp ground coriander
½ tsp cumin seeds
1 tsp ground turmeric
1 medium onion, finely
   sliced
½ medium courgette,
   grated
1 egg, beaten
3 tbsp rapeseed oil or ghee

• DAIRY-FREE
• GLUTEN-FREE
• GOOD FOR PHASE 1

1. Mix together the flour, coriander, cumin and turmeric in a bowl and season generously with salt and freshly ground black pepper. Add the onion and courgette and stir to ensure everything gets a good coating of the spicy flour, then stir in the egg.

2. Place a frying pan over a medium heat. Heat the oil or ghee, then drop heaped tablespoonfuls of the mixture into the pan, flattening them slightly and frying them for 1-2 minutes on each side, until they're crisp and golden brown. Remove them from the pan with a slotted spoon and place them on kitchen paper to drain.

Note: onions are good for your microbiome, but these may be too much of a good thing if you have IBS.

190 CALORIES

Green Banana and Pepper Stir-Fry

This is a great side dish with lots of crunch, and a slightly fruity flavour. When gently fried, unripe bananas taste more like sweet potatoes; they are more gut-friendly than potatoes, however, as the starch they contain is resistant, i.e. not rapidly converted to sugar.

Serves 4

3 tbsp olive oil

1 red onion, sliced

1 red pepper, deseeded and chopped

1 yellow pepper, deseeded and chopped

1 tsp cumin seeds

2 green bananas, sliced

Handful of fresh coriander leaves, torn

• DAIRY-FREE
• GLUTEN-FREE
• OPTION FOR PHASE 1

1. Heat the olive oil in a wok or large frying pan and sauté the onion for 2 minutes.

2. Add the peppers and cumin seeds and stir-fry for 8-10 minutes, until the peppers start to soften slightly and the onion starts to caramelise.

3. Add the banana slices and cook for a further 3-4 minutes.

4. Before serving, sprinkle the coriander and some freshly ground black pepper on top.

Note: green bananas are not ideal for IBS sufferers due to the 'scratchy' fibre they contain. For Phase 1 we suggest reducing the onion by half and replacing 1 of the peppers with 150g broccoli.

170 CALORIES

Smoky Aubergine and Cannellini Beans

Based on the Middle-Eastern dish, Baba Ganoush, this makes a wonderful side dish or dip. Those with IBS, or in the first two weeks of Phase 1, may find the fibre in it exacerbates symptoms, in which case reduce your portion size or swap the beans for chickpeas.

Serves 4 as a side dish

1 medium aubergine (about 250g)

5 tbsp olive oil

1 onion, diced

2 large garlic cloves, crushed

2 tsp fresh herbs such as thyme, parsley or oregano, chopped (or 1 tsp dried)

130g canned white beans such as haricot or cannellini (or chickpeas), drained

1 tbsp balsamic vinegar

½ tsp chilli flakes (optional)

Handful of fresh coriander, chopped

• DAIRY-FREE
• GLUTEN-FREE

1. To give the aubergine the distinctive smoky flavour, roast it whole in a wok or saucepan with the lid on, stalk still attached, with the heat on high. Allow the skin to thicken and char in places before turning it. Aim to char more than half the skin – this will take 4-5 minutes. Place it on a plate and allow it to cool. For alternative charring techniques, see tip below.

2. Using a knife, remove the stalk, then peel off and discard the skin. Dice the flesh, retaining any browned parts as these add to the flavour, and set it aside.

3. Heat the oil in a medium-sized saucepan and sauté the onion for about 5 minutes without letting it brown. Add the garlic and herbs to the pan, followed by the aubergine and beans. Mix in the balsamic vinegar and chilli to taste. Add 2-3 tbsp water to loosen the mixture.

4. Cover the pan and simmer gently for 12-15 minutes, stirring occasionally. Add 1-2 tbsp water at a time if it is drying out, to maintain a thick, creamy texture. Season it with salt and freshly ground black pepper and stir in half the coriander. Before serving, scatter the remaining coriander on top. For a more creamy texture or if you wish to serve it as a dip, blitz the mixture briefly with a hand blender.

Tip: another way to prepare the aubergine is to hold it directly over a hot flame on the cooker. Or pierce it and place it under the grill, turning it so it chars evenly. Then remove the skin as described above.

220 CALORIES

Aubergines are an excellent source of fibre and vitamins B1 and B6, as well as minerals such as potassium, copper, magnesium and manganese.

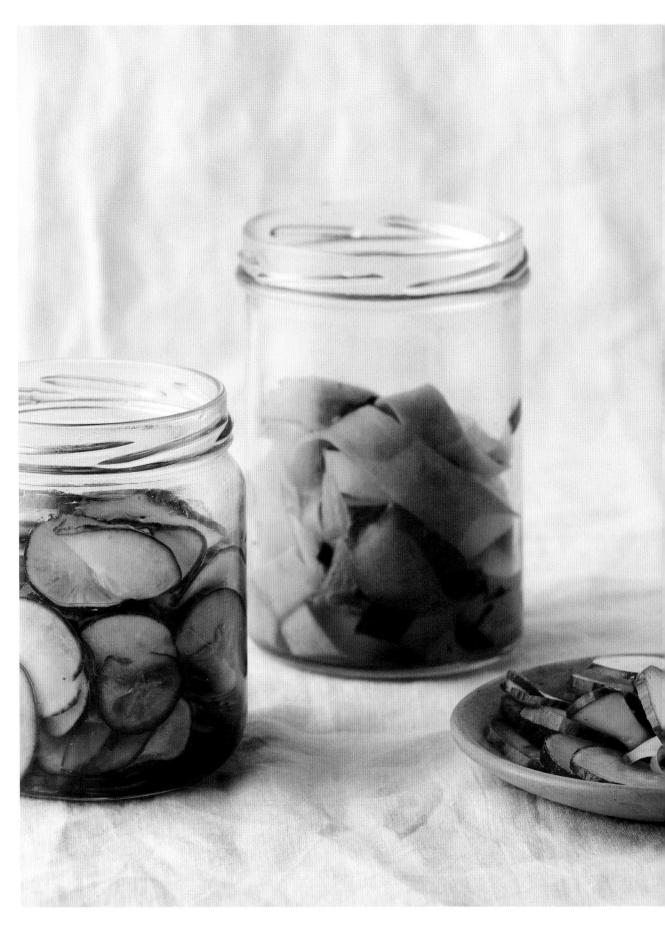

Japanese-Style Quick Pickled Veg

Finely sliced vegetables that have been lightly pickled add a delicate Japanese flavour to many dishes. Great with fish or seafood.

Serves 2

¼ cucumber

3 radishes

Generous pinch of Maldon
   sea salt

1 tsp live organic apple
   cider vinegar

1 tsp mirin wine (optional)

• DAIRY-FREE

• GLUTEN-FREE

• GOOD FOR PHASE 1

1. Slice the cucumber and radishes thinly, ideally with a mandolin, then place them in a small dish, with the salt, cider vinegar and mirin.

2. Using your fingers, massage in the salt and then leave the veg to rest for about 20 minutes.

Tips: use a Y-shaped slicer or mandolin to cut longer slices of carrot or courgette to add to the dish. For extra flavour add strips of dried nori seaweed.

20 CALORIES

Vegetable-Rich Tomato Sauce

A rich and versatile tomato sauce full of hidden goodness. Even determined vegetable avoiders are likely to enjoy it. Keep portions in the freezer ready to use.

Makes approx 1.2 litres, or 4 servings

8 tbsp olive oil

1 large onion, diced

2 garlic cloves, diced

2 celery stalks, diced

2 carrots, diced

2 medium courgettes, diced

2 red peppers, deseeded and diced

1 tbsp fresh oregano or basil, chopped (or 1 tsp dried oregano)

1 large bay leaf

½ tsp dried thyme

2 x 400g cans chopped tomatoes

425g can pumpkin purée

2 tbsp balsamic vinegar

• DAIRY-FREE
• GLUTEN-FREE
• GOOD FOR PHASE 1

1. Pour the oil into a large saucepan and sweat the onions, garlic, celery, carrots, courgettes and red peppers for 10-15 minutes over a medium heat, stirring frequently. In the last few minutes add the herbs.

2. Next add the tomatoes, pumpkin purée, vinegar and 300ml water and let the sauce simmer with the lid on for at least 30 minutes – ideally for up to an hour. You may need to top up with extra water if it is getting too thick, or remove the lid if it needs thickening.

3. When the vegetables are soft and the sauce is the desired consistency, blitz it briefly with a hand blender, leaving some chunky bits for texture. Season to taste.

Tips: you can use this tomato sauce in a variety of ways, for example as a base for meat or fish dishes, or to pour over vegetables or pasta. Change the selection of herbs to get different flavours. It also works well as a base for soup (see Spicy Lentil and Tomato Soup p62).

370 CALORIES

Puy Lentils with Balsamic Vinegar

With their uniquely peppery flavour and their ability to keep their shape and texture when cooked, Puy lentils are a cut above other lentils, containing plenty of fibre and some protein too. Delicious served hot or cold.

Serves 4
(2-4 as a side dish)

4 tbsp olive oil

1 onion, diced

1 celery stalk, diced

1 garlic clove, finely
    chopped

250g Puy lentils

2 tbsp balsamic vinegar

1 tsp fresh thyme (or ½ tsp
    dried)

450ml vegetable stock
    (or water)

Handful of fresh coriander,
    chopped

• DAIRY-FREE
• GLUTEN-FREE

1. Heat the oil in a medium-sized saucepan and sauté the onion and celery over a medium heat for 4-5 minutes, stirring occasionally. They should be soft but not browned.

2. Add the garlic and lentils and cook for another minute or so, then stir in the vinegar, thyme and stock (or water). Top up with water if needed, to cover the lentils by 1cm.

3. Bring it to the boil and leave it to simmer, covered, for 20-25 minutes, or until the lentils are firm to the bite. Season with salt and pepper and stir in the coriander before serving.

Tip: serve on a bed of salad leaves with a sprinkling of crumbled feta and sliced avocado for a light meal.

Note: the fibre in lentils can make IBS worse. Reduce your portion size, or avoid them altogether in Phase 1.

240 CALORIES

Roasted Vegetables

There is something wonderfully comforting about a tray of crispy, caramelised vegetables straight from the oven. Roasted veg also have more flavour and tend to be easier to digest.

Beets Roasted in Their Skins

Probably our favourite way of cooking beetroots, one which leaves all the goodness intact as most of the nutrients reside in the skin. They make a great accompaniment to lots of dishes.

Serves 2

175g small beetroots, scrubbed, trimmed and cut into quarters
2 tbsp olive oil
½ tsp cumin seeds
1 tbsp live apple cider vinegar
Pinch of chilli flakes to taste

• DAIRY-FREE
• GLUTEN-FREE
• GOOD FOR PHASE 1

1. Preheat the oven to 180°C/160°C fan/gas mark 4. Place the beetroot quarters in a roasting tin, then toss them in the olive oil, cumin seeds, sea salt and freshly ground black pepper.

2. Cover the tin with foil and put it in the oven for 20 minutes. Then remove the foil, drizzle over the cider vinegar and return it to the oven, uncovered, for a further 15-20 minutes or until the beets are tender and starting to brown.

3. Serve with bitter leaves, such as rocket, dandelion or baby spinach (add 10 cals).

Tip: for a more substantial meal add smoked fish, cold meats or some cheese.

150 CALORIES

Roasted Jerusalem Artichokes

Artichokes are knobbly and tedious to peel – so much easier to just give them a good scrub (thus retaining the best of the nutrients in the skin). Baked in the oven, they come out sweet and tasty, with an earthy succulence, and are loaded with gut-friendly soluble fibre, as well as iron, potassium and vitamin B1.

Serves 4

500g Jerusalem artichokes, scrubbed, and cut in half if large
2 tbsp olive oil
Juice of ½ lemon

• DAIRY-FREE
• GLUTEN-FREE

1. Preheat the oven to 180°C/160°C fan/gas mark 4. Place the artichokes in an ovenproof dish, and toss them in the olive oil and some seasoning.

2. Roast them for about 45 minutes, or until they're tender. Drizzle with the lemon juice before serving.

Roasted Purple Carrots with Tarragon

Cooking carrots, particularly with their skin still on, helps to increase the absorption of nutrients such as beta carotene; adding plenty of olive oil enhances the absorption of fat-soluble vitamins.

Serves 2

250g purple (or orange) carrots, scrubbed and trimmed
3 tbsp extra-virgin olive oil
1 tsp dried tarragon
Juice of ½ lemon

• DAIRY-FREE
• GLUTEN-FREE
• GOOD FOR PHASE 1

1. Preheat the oven to 180°C/160°C fan/gas mark 4. Place the carrots in an ovenproof dish or roasting tin. Toss them in the olive oil, tarragon and some seasoning.

2. Bake them for 20-30 minutes, stirring them occasionally, until they start to brown. Drizzle with the lemon juice before serving.

Tip: delicious served with Slow-Roast Shoulder of Lamb (page 157) or Beef and Orange Stew (page 150).

Roasted Butternut Squash

A simple, gut-friendly side dish, which boosts fibre intake and is generally very well tolerated.

Serves 2

½ small butternut squash, peeled

3 tbsp olive oil

1 tbsp Parmesan (or vegan Parmesan), grated

Juice of ½ lemon

• DAIRY-FREE
• GLUTEN-FREE
• GOOD FOR PHASE 1

1. Preheat the oven to 180°C/160°C fan/gas mark 4. Slice the butternut squash in half lengthways. Scoop out the seeds and stringy bits and cut the flesh into long slices or semicircles.

2. Spread the slices in an ovenproof dish and toss them in the olive oil and some salt and freshly ground black pepper. Bake them for 25-30 minutes, turning them occasionally.

3. Once the squash starts to brown and feels tender when pierced, sprinkle the Parmesan over it and bake it for a further 5-6 minutes. Drizzle with the lemon juice before serving.

240 CALORIES

Slow Roasted Tomatoes

Wonderful with fish, or added to a salad.

Serves 2

4 medium vine-ripened tomatoes, cut in half around the middle

2 tbsp olive oil

1 garlic clove, finely chopped

2 tsp fresh herbs, such as thyme or rosemary (or 1 tsp dried), leaves only

• DAIRY-FREE
• GLUTEN-FREE
• GOOD FOR PHASE 1

1. Preheat the oven to 120°C/100°C fan/gas mark ½.

2. Place the tomatoes in an ovenproof dish, cut side up. Drizzle with the olive oil and scatter the garlic and herbs on top. Season well.

3. Bake for 3½-4 hours, until they are soft and caramelised.

170 CALORIES

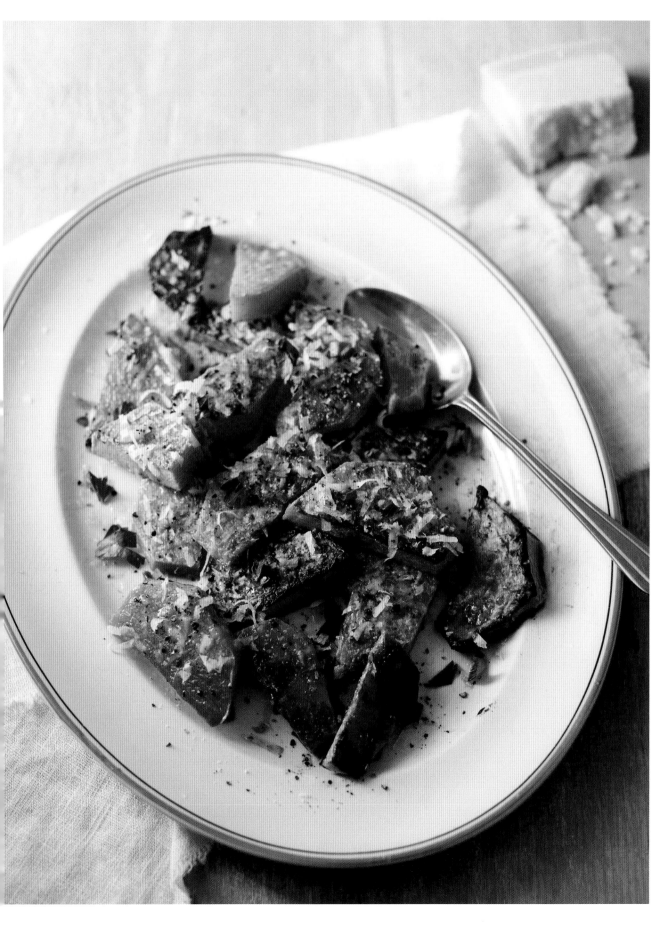

Healthy Swaps

You will have gathered by now that your gut does not thrive on foods that are sweet or starchy. Nor do these help your blood sugars or waistline, let alone your metabolism. Try some of these alternatives to potatoes, rice, pasta and noodles. There are suggestions for healthy breads in the Treats chapter, too.

Cauliflower Rice with Coriander

An ideal low-carb, gut-friendly alternative to rice to mop up the juices of a curry or a stew. Cauliflower contains some of almost every mineral and vitamin you need. And to top it all, it's high in fibre and antioxidants. Amazing that so much can be packed into such a pale and unassuming vegetable.

Serves 4
2 tbsp olive oil
1 small onion, finely
   chopped
1 small garlic clove,
   finely chopped (optional)
1 medium cauliflower
Large handful of fresh
   coriander, chopped

•DAIRY-FREE
•GLUTEN-FREE
•GOOD FOR PHASE 1

1. Heat the olive oil in a pan and sauté the onion and garlic for 4-5 minutes.

2. Meanwhile, chop the cauliflower into florets and grate it or use a food processor to turn it into 'rice'. It should look a bit like pale bulgar wheat.

3. Add the cauliflower rice to the onions and then turn up the heat and stir-fry, until it is al dente, about 6-7 minutes. Add the coriander, season and serve.

70 CALORIES

Aubergine Chips

These make a crisp, tasty and healthy alternative to starchy, sugar-spiking potato chips. Great with a light salad or to eat with a dip.

Serves 4

100g ground almonds

½ tsp cayenne pepper

1 egg

1 medium aubergine, cut into chips

3 tbsp light olive oil

• DAIRY-FREE

• GLUTEN FREE

• GOOD FOR PHASE 1

1. Preheat the oven to 200°C/180°C fan/gas mark 6. Mix the ground almonds and cayenne pepper together on a plate. Beat the egg in a bowl.

2. Dip the aubergine chips first into the egg and then into the ground almond mixture. Repeat to ensure the chips get a good even coating. Season generously with salt and freshly ground black pepper.

3. Place the chips on a greased baking tray and drizzle over the oil. Bake them for 15-20 minutes or until they're golden brown. Serve with Avocado and Lime Salsa (page 75) or one of our delicious dips (pages 72-73).

280 CALORIES

Red Rice with Resistant Starch

Red rice has the same relatively low GI as brown rice but contains extra nutrients, such as healthy polyphenols. The process of cooking then cooling the rice in the fridge for 12 hours converts some of the starchy carbohydrate into resistant starch. This gut-friendly form of fibre is not absorbed in the small intestine, but instead makes its way to the large bowel and feeds up your 'good' bacteria.

Serves 4

100g red Camargue rice

100g brown rice

1 tsp coconut oil (or mild olive oil)

• DAIRY-FREE
• GLUTEN-FREE
• GOOD FOR PHASE 1

1. Place the rice in a saucepan with a lid. Cover it with twice its volume of water and add the oil and a pinch of salt. Bring it to a boil, then allow it to simmer gently, covered, for 20-30 minutes, or until most of the water has been absorbed – at which point turn the heat off and leave it covered to steam for a further 5-10 minutes.

2. Allow the rice to cool before putting it in the fridge for 12 hours/overnight to convert more of the starch into gut-friendly resistant starch.

3. The rice is then ready to use, either cold or reheated – for example in a rice salad (page 90) or as a rice pudding (page 213). You also get the same benefit if you freeze it in portions.

Tip: you can use either red or brown rice on its own for this recipe; using both just adds a bit more texture and flavour.

90 CALORIES

Pan-Fried Courgetti Spaghetti

These days we often swap starchy spaghetti for 'courgetti' or 'noodles' made from fresh, firm vegetables such as squash or carrot. You can also go for a half-and-half version: boil a small portion of spaghetti and throw spiralised courgette into it for the last minute of cooking. Once you get a taste for it you will probably find you abandon the spaghetti altogether.

Serves 2

2 tbsp olive oil

2 large courgettes,
   spiralised

1 small garlic clove,
   crushed (optional)

Squeeze of lemon

• DAIRY-FREE

• GLUTEN FREE

• GOOD FOR PHASE 1

1. Place a large frying pan over a medium heat. Add the oil and fry the courgetti with the garlic for 1-1½ minutes, stirring frequently. It needs to remain al dente, so don't overcook or it will become soggy.

2. Season it with Maldon sea salt, freshly ground black pepper and a squeeze of lemon, and serve it immediately with a main dish, such as Turkey and Mushroom Bolognese (page 131) or Vegetable-Rich Tomato Sauce (page 168).

130 CALORIES

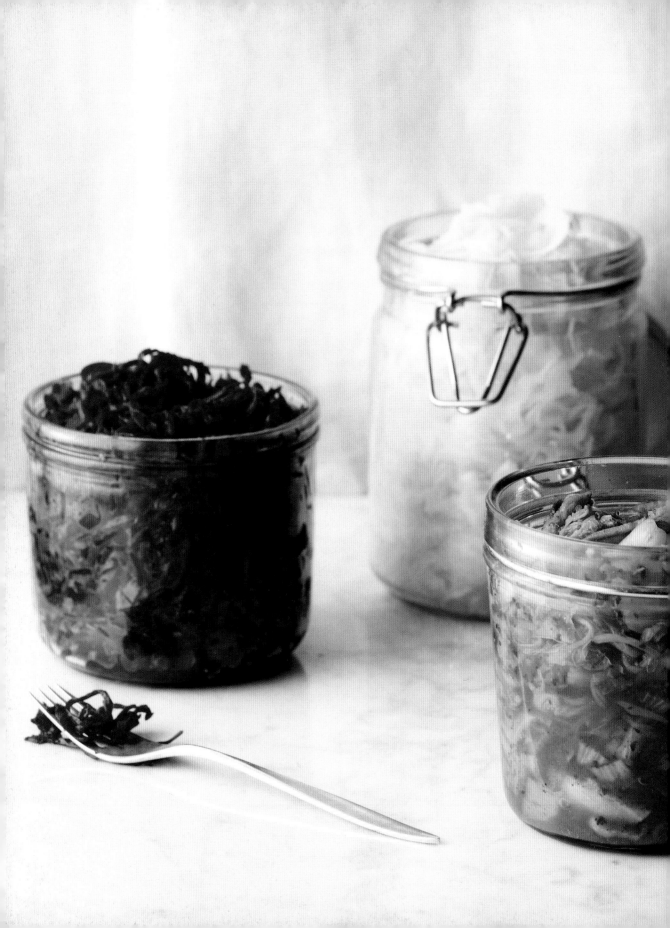

FERMENTS

Fermenting is making a come-back in
kitchens around the world – and for
good reason. It's cheap, it's fun and
there is hardly a better way of nurturing
the good guys in your gut. We should
all have some jars of interesting things
fizzing away on the worktop.

Kombucha

Kombucha is a form of fermented tea which has been brewed for millennia in China, Russia and Eastern Europe. It makes a refreshing drink with a subtle apple flavour and a sweet and sour fizz. It is produced by a living organism, or 'mother', known as a Symbiotic Culture of Bacteria and Yeast (or SCOBY), a complex culture of micro-organisms which acts as a probiotic providing your gut with healthy microbes.

Kombucha is an easy and forgiving ferment to manage. First you need to source your SCOBY – you can buy them online (see cleverguts.com). It looks somewhat like a squashed beige jellyfish and floats like a rubbery raft on or in the tea, protecting and maintaining the fermentation. To encourage the aerobic process, the brew needs to be open to fresh air. The recipe below is for a relatively low-sugar version. Calorie counts are not included as much of the sugar added is used up in the fermentation process. How much remains depends on how many days you ferment it for.

Makes 1 litre

A SCOBY

1 litre spring or filtered water (tap water contains chlorine which can prevent fermentation)

2-3 teabags, ideally organic black, green or white tea. Your kombucha will probably prefer some teas to others as each SCOBY is unique (see page 182)

60g unbleached sugar

You will also need:

1 litre wide-mouth glass jar

1 litre glass bottle with tight-fitting lid

Small piece of cloth or muslin

• DAIRY-FREE

• GLUTEN-FREE

1. Place your SCOBY, along with the fluid it is floating in, in a clean 1 litre jar. Empty the kettle and pour in about 300ml filtered water, bring it to the boil, then pour it into a 1 litre jug containing the teabags. Add the sugar and allow it to steep for 30 minutes. Remove the teabags and pour in the remaining water to make it up to almost 1 litre of sweetened tea.

2. Once the tea is at room temperature you can add it to the jar with the SCOBY. If it is too hot it will kill the SCOBY. The water level in the jar needs to remain at least 2cm below the top of the jar. Cover it with a clean piece of moderately tightly woven cloth, to keep out dust and bugs yet still allow air flow. Muslin is not quite densely woven enough, though you could use 2 or 3 layers of it. Secure the cloth with an elastic band. Don't use a lid as it needs the air. Then leave it to brew on the kitchen surface out of direct sunlight at room temperature.

3. After a few days you will notice small bubbles forming around the edge of the SCOBY. Your alien life form is springing into action! If you lift the cloth you will notice a delicious sweet, slightly tart smell. Pale brownish stringy floaty bits will probably accumulate below the SCOBY and the liquid may become a bit cloudy. That's fine.

4. It will be ready to drink after around 5 days but can be brewed for longer according to taste, as it develops a richer, tarter flavour with a slight fizz. Use a clean spoon to taste a little. It is probably best decanted well within 2 weeks. The longer it is left, the more vinegary and fizzy it becomes.

5. When it's ready, decant the liquid into a clean glass bottle with a tight lid. Leave behind roughly the same volume of fluid as the size of the SCOBY, so it can be restarted in the next few days by adding more sweetened tea to repeat the cycle. Place the bottle in the fridge, leaving only about 1cm air under the lid, to halt the aerobic process and prevent further fermenting. This also helps to stop it turning to vinegar (though you can use this in cooking). As it is a live ferment, the container might burst or leak if it is left in a warm place.

Tips: though kombucha is usually well tolerated, we suggest starting with a small glass so you can introduce it to your gut gradually. Some people prefer to drink it diluted with water.

Only use black or green tea that has come from the tea plant, *Camellia sinensis.* Herbal infusions are not technically tea; they are simply herbs or fruits infused in boiling water (this includes rooibos tea). When we added a peppermint teabag to a second brew, the SCOBY went mouldy and had to be discarded. Some cultures thrive better on one type of tea than another, depending on what it was originally grown in. So, if you have a spare SCOBY, experiment and see what works for yours. Green tea is a particularly popular flavour and may have extra health benefits too.

Don't store the SCOBY in the fridge. It may survive for short periods but the cold will weaken it and it may take time to recover, or not recover at all. You should of course store the bottled kombucha in the fridge.

It is not thriving if you see patches of black mould or if it smells unpleasant, rancid or 'cheesy'. If this happens, sadly you will need to discard it and start again.

If you are away for a few weeks: simply make a fresh batch and leave it to do its own thing. You may find that it has turned to vinegar on your return but the SCOBY will be fine. Decant most of the fluid as usual, then top it up again with fresh sweet tea.

Managing the SCOBY: over a matter of weeks the SCOBY will gradually get thicker, more uniform in shape and float on top. When it has grown to 1-2cm thickness you can split it to make 2 thinner disks or cut a chunk off it. Remove the extra disk and place it in a jar along with at least twice its volume in fluid from the 'mother'. This can be kept as a spare, just in case, or to pass on to other 'boochas' to grow their own.

Storing kombucha: when a spare kombucha has been allowed to rest, you need to add 40-50g sugar every 4-6 weeks to keep it alive and ticking over. Then every 2-3 months, discard most of the liquid in your kombucha 'hotel' and top up the jar to four-fifths with fresh sweet tea to keep it going.

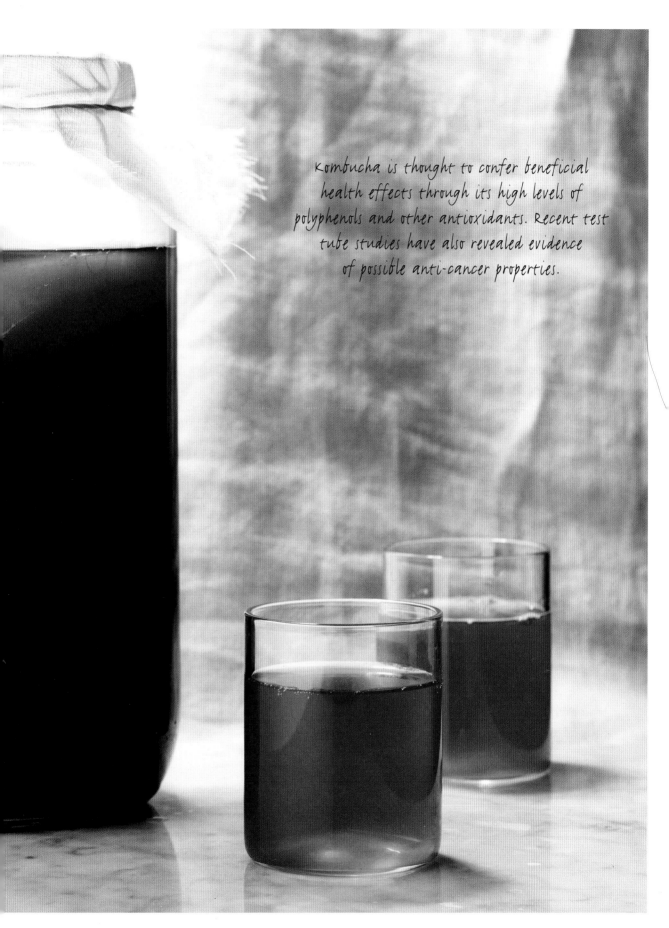

Kombucha is thought to confer beneficial health effects through its high levels of polyphenols and other antioxidants. Recent test tube studies have also revealed evidence of possible anti-cancer properties.

Preserved Lemons

Lemon peel contains twice the amount of vitamins of lemon flesh, and has a more intense flavour than the juice, with a hint of bitterness. Once fermented, the flavours mellow and the peel softens. Preserved lemons work brilliantly in small quantities in both sweet and savoury dishes (such as Easy Chicken Tagine, page 127, Lemony Buttermilk Dressing, page 118, or Cauliflower Baked with Lemon and Almonds, page 95). The majority of shop-bought versions are devoid of live bacteria, and in our experience can have an industrial mouthwash taste to them. So it is well worth making your own…

6-7 large unwaxed lemons, preferably organic
1 tbsp live apple cider vinegar
1 heaped tbsp Maldon sea salt
½ tsp coriander seeds (optional)

You will also need:
250ml glass jar with well-fitting lid

• DAIRY-FREE
• GLUTEN-FREE
• GOOD FOR PHASE 1

1. Wash the lemons. Cut them in half and squeeze some of the juice from each into the jar. Then cut the halves in half again. Slice each lemon quarter finely, discarding the seeds and some of the pith.

2. Pack the slices tightly into the jar, scattering a generous pinch of salt between the layers until it is used up.

3. Use a wooden spoon or the end of a rolling pin to squash the lemon slices down and force out the air bubbles. There should be enough juice to cover them. If necessary, top up with salted filtered or spring water, using 1 heaped tsp sea salt to 200ml water. As it's an anaerobic process, prevent contact with the air by covering the surface with a small dish or a boiled clean pebble before closing the jar.

4. For the first few days you need to 'burp' the lemons a couple of times a day to release any trapped bubbles produced by fermentation. This means pressing them down so that they are always submerged. Leave them to ferment at room temperature for between 5 days and 2 weeks. Then store them in the fridge to prevent further fermentation.

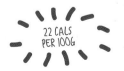

22 CALS PER 100G

Red Cabbage Sauerkraut

This crunchy, dark-red sauerkraut is one of our favourites. As well as the wonderful burst of colour it brings to a meal, it has an appealing sweet and sour flavour. What's more, it's packed with those healthy phytonutrients found in pigmented veg. It can be used with almost any food, including for breakfast…

Makes 1 litre

1 small red cabbage (about 1kg), core and outer leaves removed, chopped

2 medium onions (about 200g) chopped

4 tsp Maldon sea salt

1 tsp mustard seeds

1 tsp coriander seeds, toasted

½ -1 tsp chilli flakes

You will also need:

1 litre glass jar with well-fitting lid

• DAIRY-FREE
• GLUTEN-FREE

1. In a large bowl, massage the salt into the cabbage and onion and leave them to sweat for 1-2 hours. The liquid from the veg will collect in the bottom of the bowl. Reserve it for later.

2. Transfer the salted veg to the glass jar, cramming them in with clean hands or the end of a wooden rolling pin. Pour in the reserved liquid from the bowl and push the veg firmly down again. The liquid should rise above the surface.

3. If there is not enough liquid, even after a few hours, you can top up with brine made with 1 tsp Maldon sea salt dissolved in 200ml filtered water. The water level should be ½-1cm above the veg and about 2½cm below the top of the jar. Place a stone, ceramic or glass object on top of the veg to keep them submerged.

4. Leave the sauerkraut to stand on the counter top out of direct sunlight for 3-14 days, depending on the room temperature and how the taste is developing. Test it regularly for flavour. Then store it in a sealed jar in the fridge. It will keep for a few months.

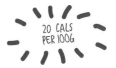

20 CALS PER 100G

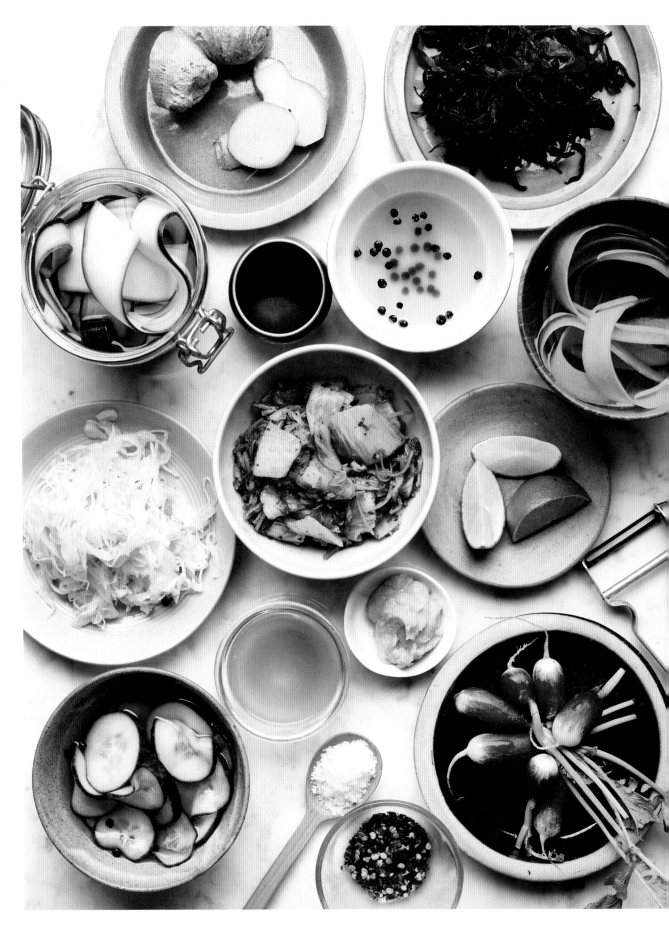

Vegetable Ferments

Once you get going, the principles of fermentation are simple and you can start working with all sorts of different vegetables.

Makes 1 litre

1kg tough veg, such as cabbage, beetroot, onions radishes or carrots, or a mixture of all, finely sliced
4-5 tsp Maldon sea salt
Flavouring, such as 1 tsp mustard seeds, fennel seeds, coriander seeds, chilli flakes or peppercorns, and herbs, such as a small bunch of dill, a sprig of rosemary or 1-2 bay leaves

You will also need:
1 litre glass jar with well-fitting lid

• DAIRY-FREE
• GLUTEN-FREE

Massage and press the ingredients together in a large bowl, scattering salt over as you go. Then transfer them to the jar and press them down firmly with the end of a rolling pin or wooden spoon, leaving 2½cm space at the top of the jar. Let them rest for 30-60 minutes, to allow the salt to draw the liquid out of them.

The veg need to be kept submerged, as it is an anaerobic process. Place a heavy object on the surface, such as a clean boiled pebble or a glass dish to prevent contact with the air. If there isn't enough liquid to cover the veg make extra brine by dissolving 1 tsp salt in 200ml filtered water. (Tap water contains chlorine which kills the bacteria.) Seal the jar tightly. Leave it at room temperature, away from direct sunlight.

For the first 3-4 days the veg need to be 'burped' a couple of times a day, to release the gases that are a by-product of fermentation. Press down on the veg using a wooden spoon or the end of a rolling pin to release trapped bubbles. Taste them occasionally. They gradually get sweeter and softer. When they are ready – soft with a bit of crunch (after 5-14 days) – place the sealed jar in the fridge to prevent further fermentation. The veg will keep for a few months.

You can vary the fermentation by changing the kind of veg (or fruit) used, or by altering the saltiness. By adding different seasonings and seeds, you can also change the flavours. Be creative and try different combinations.

Pickled Courgettes with Mustard Seeds

Pickling is a traditional way of preserving vegetables and fruit at a time of plenty. Sadly, the word is now associated with sterile items that you pull off the supermarket shelves, almost certainly containing few live micro-organisms. This pickle goes with most meals – try it with Black Bean Beet Burgers (page 147), or fish. Or simply nibble on it before a meal to get those digestive juices flowing.

Makes 500ml

300g mini courgettes, topped and tailed, sliced in half lengthways

½ small white onion, sliced

2 tsp Maldon sea salt, plus ½ tbsp for the brine

1 tsp mustard seeds

1 tsp coriander seeds

½ tsp chilli flakes

Small pinch of black tea leaves

You will also need:

500ml glass jar with well-fitting lid

• DAIRY-FREE
• GLUTEN-FREE

1. Wash the courgettes under the tap and rinse them with filtered water to remove any remaining chlorine. Place them on a large plate cut side up and scatter the onion on top, followed by the salt. Leave them for 1-2 hours, until the salt has drawn the water out.

2. Toast the mustard and coriander seeds in a hot pan for a minute or two, to bring out the flavour. Put them in the jar, along with the chilli flakes and the tea (the tannin in the tea helps the veg to remain firm).

3. Add the veg to the jar, along with the liquid and any salt left on the plate. Tilt the jar slightly so the courgettes are packed standing upright.

4. Dissolve ½ tbsp salt in 250ml filtered water. Pour this over the courgettes so that they're covered with about 1cm liquid. Place a small glass or ceramic object on top to keep them submerged. If they dry out, top the jar up with brine made with 1 tsp salt to 200ml filtered water.

5. Stand the jar on the counter top out of direct sunlight or excessive heat for 2-5 days. I prefer the veg after 2-3 days as they remain slightly more crunchy. Over the first 3 days or so, open the lid daily to release the fermentation gases. If it is active, you will see tiny bubbles forming as lactic acid ferments the sugars in the veg. When the pickle is ready, store it in the fridge. It will keep for 2-3 weeks.

30 CALS PER 100G

Spicy Pickled Onions

Most pickled onion recipes seem to involve pouring boiling-hot vinegar and/
or brine mixtures over the onions, which kills all the natural *Lactobacilli*
and other micro-organisms needed for fermentation and the production of
probiotics. In this recipe, they are lightly pickled in microbiome-friendly cider
vinegar. The result is a beautifully sweet, spicy pickle, which is great sliced
and scattered on a salad, or nibbled with cheese.

Makes 350ml
½ tsp peppercorns
½ tsp coriander seeds
½ tsp mustard seeds
Pinch of chilli flakes
(optional)
300-350g shallots, or any
small onions, peeled,
topped and tailed
200ml live apple cider
vinegar

You will also need:
350ml glass jar with well-
fitting lid

• DAIRY-FREE
• GLUTEN-FREE

1. Toast the coriander seeds in a hot pan for a minute
or two to bring out the flavour, then put them in the jar
with the other spices.

2. Cut the larger shallots or onions in half and add
them to the jar until it is just over three-quarters full.

3. Dilute the cider vinegar by mixing it with 100ml
filtered water. Pour this into the jar – there should be
about 1cm liquid above the onions. Place a small glass
or ceramic object on top to keep them submerged.

4. Leave them to ferment for 3-14 days. Taste them
regularly and, when you're happy with them, pop them
in the fridge to prevent further fermentation. They
will keep for 3-4 weeks. Drain or rinse off the vinegar
before serving.

20 CALS
PER 100G

Kefir Milk

Kefir is a fermented milk drink that tastes like a tangy, runny yoghurt. The culture is grown either from powder or, more commonly, 'grains', which look like tiny soft cauliflower florets. These contain a complex ecosystem of as many as 40-50 types of bacteria and yeasts, which work together to produce one of the most probiotic-rich drinks available.

Makes 1 litre
1 litre organic full-fat milk
Kefir starter powder
  or grains

You will also need:
1 litre glass container
  with lid (or cover with
  clingfilm)

•GLUTEN-FREE

Kefir starter cultures. These are usually available as fresh grains or as dried powder in sachets. If you are lucky, you might be given fresh grains by a friend who has cultivated an excess. They can be reused repeatedly. Our kefir culture has been producing about a litre of kefir a week for some months now. You can also buy the cultures from health shops or online (or go to cleverguts.com).

Kefir is best fermented between 22 and 24°C, over about 24 hours. It sets more quickly when warmer and can take up to 30 hours on a cold day. Avoid stirring it while it is fermenting.

If using fresh grains, add 2 tbsp for 500ml organic full-fat milk. Drop them into the bottom of the jar and stir well. Leave it in a warm place.

If using powder, follow the instructions on the pack, which are generally as follows: pour 100ml of the milk into a container and mix with the powder to form a smooth paste. Then add the rest of the milk and stir for at least 5 minutes. (If you wish to produce more batches of kefir you can make up a bag of powder, a bit like a bouquet garni. To do this cut a circle of clean muslin about 10cm in diameter and pour the powdered kefir into the centre. Tie it into a bundle with a clean piece of string and place it in the base of the jar before adding the milk. Stir gently for 5 minutes to disperse some of the powder through the milk.)

The kefir milk is ready when it is lightly set.
At this point, scooping a spoonful out will leave a small indent in the surface. Once it has been stirred it looks like thin curdled milk. Strain all the contents through a fine nylon sieve into a 1 litre jug. Use a spoon to gently scoop up the small grainy jellied lumps left in the sieve. Place the creamy kefir liquid in a covered glass jug or a bowl in the fridge to keep cool.

Keep the grains. These can be stored in a clean container in the fridge for a few days, just covered with kefir milk, until you are ready to top up with more milk and start the next batch of fermentation. If you get in the flow, after a month or two you will have more grains or a fuller muslin bag than you need. These can then be split, stored in the fridge or given away to create another colony.

If using powder in a bundle, it should be discarded after a couple of months.

70 CALORIES PER 100ML

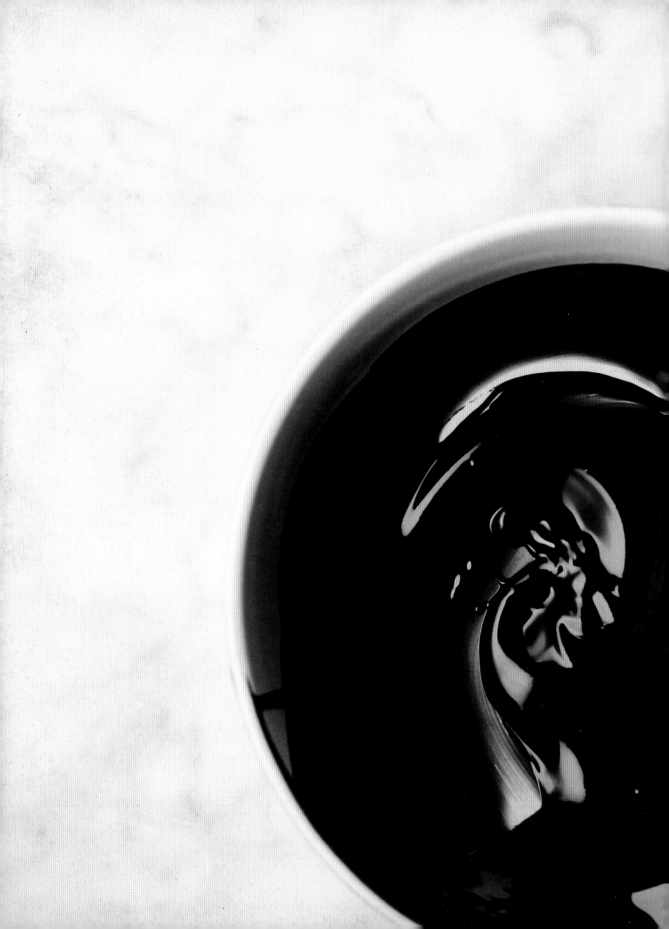

TREATS

Go for 'good' treats which include a strong dose of healthy fibre and are relatively low in sugar. If you have a sweet tooth it can take time to reset your taste buds. Stick with it – they will soon come back to life.

Breads

These breads are either gluten-free, or made with grains containing little gluten compared to that found in modern wheat. There is also a fermented sourdough, a traditional form of bread which the gut tolerates relatively well. Try them for breakfast with butter, Marmite and scrambled eggs. Or enjoy them with Nut Butter (page 123), or a dollop of cream cheese and a spoonful of Strawberry Chia 'Jam' (page 208). Just not too often!

Mug Bread

Instant, fresh, gluten-free and delicious.

Makes 4 small round slices
2 tsp coconut oil
1 large egg
2 tbsp ground almonds or ground walnuts
3 tbsp ground flaxseeds
½ tsp baking powder
Generous pinch of salt

• DAIRY-FREE
• GLUTEN-FREE

1. Microwave the coconut oil in a mug with straight sides for 20-30 seconds on high, then use it to grease the sides of the mug.

2. In a small bowl, thoroughly mix together the egg, 2 tsp water, the nuts, ground flaxseeds, baking powder and salt. Pour the mixture into the mug and stir with a fork to incorporate the coconut oil, making sure the top is level.

3. Microwave for 1 minute on high. If the bread still appears very moist, microwave for another 10-20 seconds. Avoid overcooking as this will make it rubbery.

4. Tip the bread out of the cup – it may need loosening with a knife. If it is still runny at the bottom, put it back in the cup and microwave it on high for a further 10-20 seconds.

5. Allow it to cool for a few minutes on its side, then cut it into slices.

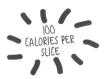
100 CALORIES PER SLICE

Wholemeal Flatbread

Flatbreads are easy to make and ideal for mopping up sauces and eating with dips and salads. Unfortunately, shop-bought white-flour flatbreads and chapattis tend to have a disastrous impact on blood sugars, driving weight gain and type 2 diabetes. This wholemeal version will be absorbed more slowly and cause less of a blood sugar spike. The fibre will also nurture your good gut bacteria.

Makes 4

250g wholemeal flour,
   such as spelt (or use
   wholegrain buckwheat or
   besan flour as a gluten-
   free option)
120ml cold water
40ml olive oil
1 tsp baking powder
1 tsp salt and a grinding of
   black pepper

• DAIRY-FREE
• GLUTEN-FREE OPTION

1. Mix all the ingredients in a bowl to form a dough. Knead it briefly on a surface dusted with flour. Cover it and leave it to rest for 30 minutes.

2. Divide the dough into 4 and roll the pieces into flat rounds approximately 10mm thick on a lightly floured work surface. To prevent bubbles forming pierce each one a few times with a fork.

3. Heat a griddle or large frying pan and cook 1 flatbread at a time for 1-3 minutes. When it starts to brown, turn it over and cook it for 1-2 minutes on the other side. If a bubble appears, press it down gently to release the steam.

4. Serve the flatbreads warm, or cool them on a rack.

Note: spelt is an ancient grain related to wheat but one which contains relatively lower amounts of gluten.

310 CALORIES

Seeded Soda Bread

A crispy loaf with added crunch and flavour thanks to the toasted seeds. This is another easy bread which doesn't require much kneading. The mildly acidic buttermilk or kefir reacts with the rising agent (bicarbonate of soda) to produce carbon dioxide which creates the bubbles and does the leavening.

Makes 1 good-sized loaf
(about 10 slices)

200g wholegrain
  buckwheat flour
100g plain white flour
  (or gluten-free flour)
1 tsp bicarbonate of soda
35g sunflower seeds
25g sesame seeds
25g ground linseeds
25g chia seeds
1 tbsp maple syrup
160ml kefir (or buttermilk)
A little milk for brushing

•GLUTEN-FREE OPTION

1. Preheat the oven to 200°C/180°C fan/gas mark 6. In a bowl, mix together the flours, bicarbonate of soda and two-thirds of the seeds. Make a well in the centre and pour in the maple syrup and kefir and mix everything together to form a soft dough.

2. Turn the dough out on to a floured work surface and gently knead it. Make a round loaf and place it on a floured baking sheet. Cut a cross in the top with a sharp knife.

3. Brush the surface with a little milk, then sprinkle the remaining seeds over the top, pressing them in slightly. Bake the loaf for 30-35 minutes, until it sounds hollow when tapped underneath. Leave it to cool on a wire rack. It can be frozen on the day of baking.

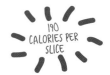
190 CALORIES PER SLICE

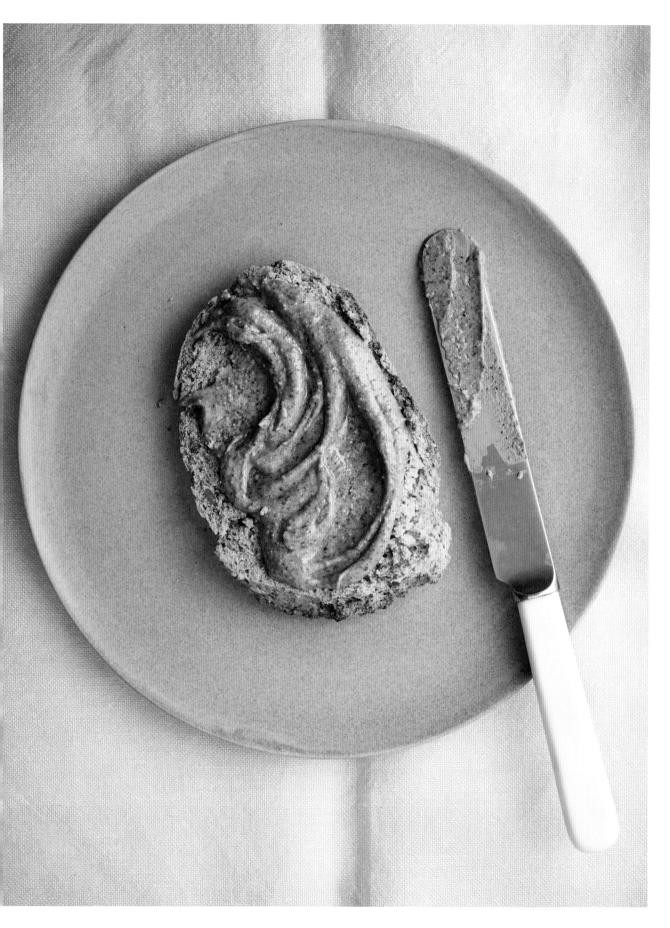

No-Knead Sourdough

Sourdough is a method of breadmaking that involves a fermentation process using naturally occurring *Lactobacilli* and yeast. The bread rises slowly and as a result maintains a more complex carbohydrate structure, producing a firmer loaf. The fermentation also appears to break down some of the gluten in the flour, making it easier on the gut than other bread.

Thanks to Judith Starling aka The Wild Baker for this recipe – her simple approach helps to demystify what seems like a complicated process. It is important to remember that the taste relies on many things – temperature, flour, weather, fermentation, time. This recipe uses kamut flour, an ancient grain that is high in protein and gives great depth of flavour. But you can use any strong wholemeal flour.

Here we assume you have a sourdough starter. You'll find more information on cleverguts.com, including how to source it online. You can make your own starter in a traditional way by using the 'wild' yeast and *Lactobacilli* present in flour. Mix a small amount with water to produce the 'mother', and then 'feed' it with a tbsp each of flour and water over the next 3-5 days. Some people add a spoonful of live buttermilk or yoghurt to help get the process underway.

Makes 1 large loaf, about about 10 slices

2 tbsp starter

445g strong white flour, or gluten-free option

95g strong wholemeal flour, or gluten-free option

150g kamut flour (or wholemeal or gluten-free flour)

1 tbsp olive oil

Strong white flour for dusting

2 tbsp semolina or gluten-free flour for dusting

•DAIRY-FREE

•GLUTEN-FREE OPTION

•GOOD FOR PHASE 1

The morning of the day before you want to bake your loaf, remove your starter from the fridge and feed it with 25g strong white flour, 25g strong wholemeal flour and 50g water. Cover it with clingfilm and leave it to prove all day at room temperature.

In the evening you should see bubbles forming on the surface or that the starter has risen, or both. Place the starter in a bowl and stir in 70g strong white flour and 70g strong wholemeal flour and 110g water – it should have a fairly thick consistency. Cover it with clingfilm and leave it overnight. It should be clearly fermenting – thick, sticky and bubbly. This is your 'pre-ferment'.

The next day, take 250g of the pre-ferment out of the bowl and place the remainder in a Kilner jar in the fridge – this will become the starter for your next loaf. Add 275ml tepid water, 150g kamut flour, 350g strong white flour and the salt to the pre-ferment in the bowl. Mix the ingredients together with your hands (or in a food processor with a dough hook or a bread maker), until you have a smooth soft dough. Oil a bowl and place the dough in it and cover it with lightly oiled clingfilm. Leave it for at least 5-6 hours at room temperature – the dough will only rise a small amount – 50% is fine.

Once it has risen, remove it from the bowl and on a very lightly floured work surface, bring the edges of the dough to the centre in a circular pattern, making a rounded loaf, and causing tension on the underside. Place the dough, seam side up, in a proving basket dusted with a small amount of flour to prevent sticking, or use a bowl lined with a tea towel, dusted with flour. Cover it again with oiled clingfilm and leave it to rise at room temperature for 1-3 hours.

Preheat the oven to the hottest temperature and place a baking tray inside to heat up. Just before you are ready to bake the loaf, place a roasting tin of boiling water in the bottom of the oven (this helps to create steam). Sprinkle the semolina over the hot baking tray (or use a sheet of reusable non-stick baking paper or silicone). Turn the loaf out on to the baking tray and quickly slash the top with a sharp knife before putting it in the oven. Bake it at 250°C/230°C fan/gas mark 10 for 10 minutes, then reduce the temperature to 190°C/170°C fan/gas mark 5 for 35-40 minutes. The loaf is cooked if it sounds hollow when tapped underneath. Rest it on a wire rack to cool before slicing it.

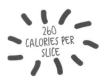

260
CALORIES PER
SLICE

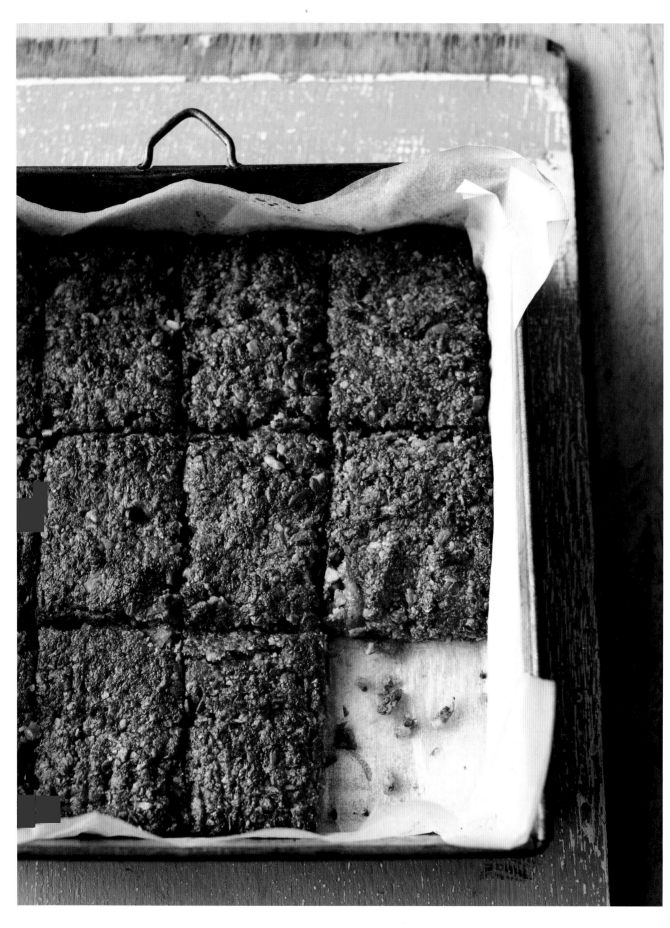

Healthy Nutrient Bars and Cakes

We would encourage you to avoid snacks between meals as this brief period of 'fasting' gives your body time to repair itself. As soon as you snack, any fat-burning stops and your good gut bacteria, such as *Akkermansia*, abandon their vital job of repairing the protective mucous lining of the gut wall. If you do yearn for a snack, it is best enjoyed after lunch, not only because it is digested more slowly after a meal, reducing the sugar spike, but also because you are likely to be moving around then and therefore burning the calories.

Apricot and Pistachio Bars

A tangy bar with crunchy nuts which your microbiome will love. These will keep your energy levels balanced for hours.

Makes 12
80g pitted dates, diced
Grated zest and juice
  of 1 orange
80g dried apricots, diced
75g coconut oil
160g pistachios
Seeds from 2
  cardamom pods
2 tbsp ground flaxseeds
¼ tsp salt

• DAIRY-FREE
• GLUTEN-FREE

1. Preheat the oven to 180°C/160°C fan/gas mark 4. Line a 20cm square tin with baking paper.

2. Soften the dates by gentling heating them in the orange juice in a small saucepan for 2 minutes. Remove the pan from the heat and add the apricots and coconut oil.

3. Blitz the pistachios and cardamom seeds in a food processor or with a hand blender until you have a coarse crumb. Add the date mixture and ground flaxseeds and pulse again.

4. Spoon the mixture into the tin, spreading it evenly to the edges. Bake it for 20-25 minutes, until it is just starting to brown on top. Remove it from the oven and allow it to cool slightly in the tin before cutting it into 12 bars. Store the bars in an airtight container for up to 5 days.

190 CALORIES

Chocolate Aubergine Cake with Pear and Walnuts

Serves 8

1 medium aubergine
  skin on, diced
150g dark chocolate (min.
  70% cocoa solids), broken
  into pieces
60g coconut oil
60g pitted dates, chopped
½ tsp salt
3 eggs, beaten
1 tsp baking powder
80g ground almonds
  (or 100g gluten-free
  brown flour)
80g walnuts, chopped
1½ pears, cubed

• DAIRY-FREE
• GLUTEN-FREE OPTION

1. Preheat the oven to 180°C/160°C fan/gas mark 4. Grease and line a 20cm cake tin with baking paper.

2. Steam the aubergine for 15 minutes or until it is soft. Then place it, still hot, in a bowl. Immediately add the chocolate and coconut oil and stir until they have more or less melted. Then mix in the chopped dates.

3. Blitz with a hand blender to obtain a smooth paste. Add the salt, eggs, baking powder and ground almonds and whizz one more time, then stir the walnuts and pears into the mixture.

4. Spoon the mixture into the prepared tin and bake it for 35-40 minutes, until a knife inserted into the centre comes out clean. Leave it to cool in the tin for 10 minutes, then transfer it to a wire rack.

370
CALORIES

Chocolate and Walnut Bites

Makes 16

200g walnuts
100g pecan nuts
75g sultanas or raisins
225g pitted dates
55g cacao powder
65g coconut oil, melted
90g rolled oats (or GF)
20g desiccated coconut
½ tsp ground cinnamon
2 tbsp cacao nibs

• DAIRY-FREE
• GLUTEN-FREE OPTION

1. Grease and line a 20cm loose-bottomed square tin with baking paper. Place the walnuts, pecans and sultanas in a bowl and cover them with boiling water. Leave them to soak for 15 minutes, then drain them and blitz them in a food processor. Add the dates and blend again, then tip in the cacao, coconut oil, oats, desiccated coconut and ground cinnamon and process again until everything is well combined.

2. Press the mixture into the prepared tin, spreading it evenly with the back of a spoon and ensuring that it is level. Lightly press the cacao nibs into the surface, and chill the mixture for at least 2 hours before cutting it into 16 bars.

280
CALORIES

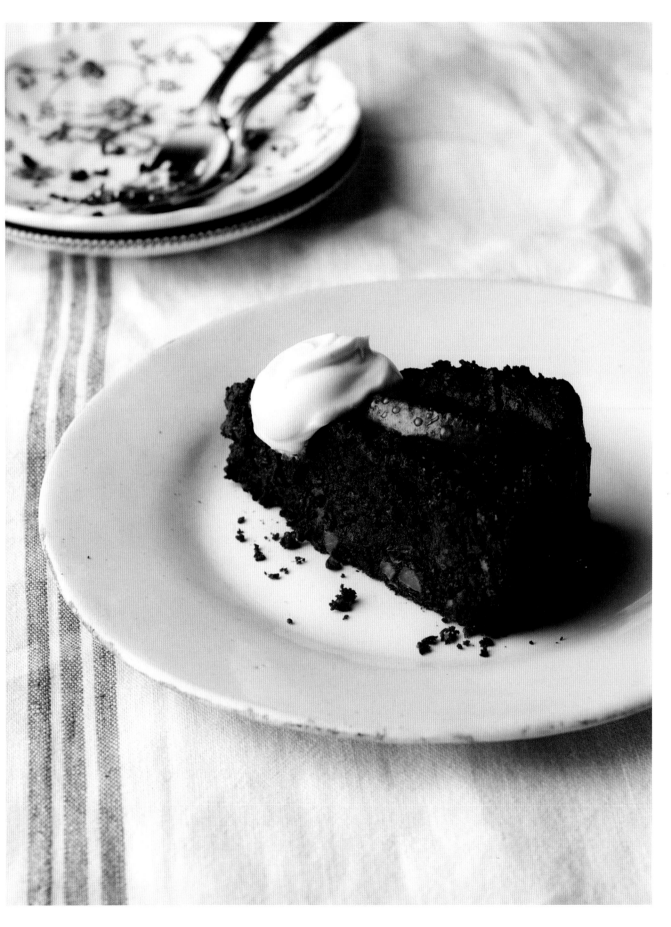

Pistachio and Olive Oil Cake

A mouth-watering cake celebrating the harmonious combination of green pistachios and olive oil.

Serves 12

100g dried apricots, chopped

Grated zest and juice of ½ lemon

2 eggs

3 tbsp extra-virgin olive oil

60g coconut oil, melted

120g shelled pistachios

70g ground almonds

1 tsp baking powder

Pinch of salt

1 tbsp honey or maple syrup

•DAIRY-FREE
•GLUTEN-FREE

1. Preheat the oven to 160°C/140°C fan/gas mark 3. Lightly grease an 18cm square cake tin. Place the chopped apricots in a small saucepan along with the lemon zest and juice and 1 tbsp water. Cover the pan and simmer gently for a few minutes to soften the apricots, then remove them from the heat and allow them to cool.

2. Whisk the eggs in a bowl, then stir in the olive oil, coconut oil and apricots.

3. Blitz 100g of the pistachios in a food processor, add the ground almonds, baking powder and salt and pulse again. Finally, pour in the egg mixture and honey and blend everything together.

4. Tip the mixture into the cake tin, crush the remaining pistachios and sprinkle them on top. Bake the cake in the oven for 25-28 minutes until it's golden on top and a knife inserted in the centre comes out fairly clean. Leave it to rest in the tin for 10 minutes, then turn it out to cool on a wire rack.

200 CALORIES

Exotic Carrot Cake

Another deliciously moist vegetable- and nut-based cake. It doesn't melt instantly in your mouth and spike your sugars, but gives you a bit more to chew on, leaving enough fibre to reach your microbiome. The cardamom adds a wonderful, exotic aroma.

Serves 12

320g carrots, grated

80g dates, finely chopped
  (or 1 tbsp honey)

3 large eggs

150g coconut oil

Zest of 1 orange

Seeds from 8 cardamom
  pods

160g wholemeal buckwheat
  flour (or gluten-free flour)

120g desiccated coconut,
  reserving 1 tbsp for
  scattering on top

1 tbsp baking powder

½ tsp salt

120g chopped walnuts

• DAIRY-FREE
• GLUTEN-FREE

1. Preheat the oven to 170°C/150°C fan/gas mark 3½. Grease and line a 20cm cake tin with baking paper.

2. Mix together the carrots, dates, eggs, coconut oil and orange zest in a large bowl, then stir in the rest of the ingredients, except the walnuts. Blitz the mixture briefly with a hand blender or in a food processor, then vigorously stir in the nuts.

3. Pour the mixture into the prepared cake tin and bake it in the centre of the oven for 60-75 minutes. It is cooked when a knife inserted in the centre comes out clean. If the top is browning before the centre is done, cover it with a piece of foil.

4. Scatter 1 tbsp desiccated coconut on the surface of the cake 5 minutes before removing it from the oven.

Tip: once the pack of desiccated coconut is opened, keep it sealed in the freezer so it stays sweet and fresh.

350 CALORIES

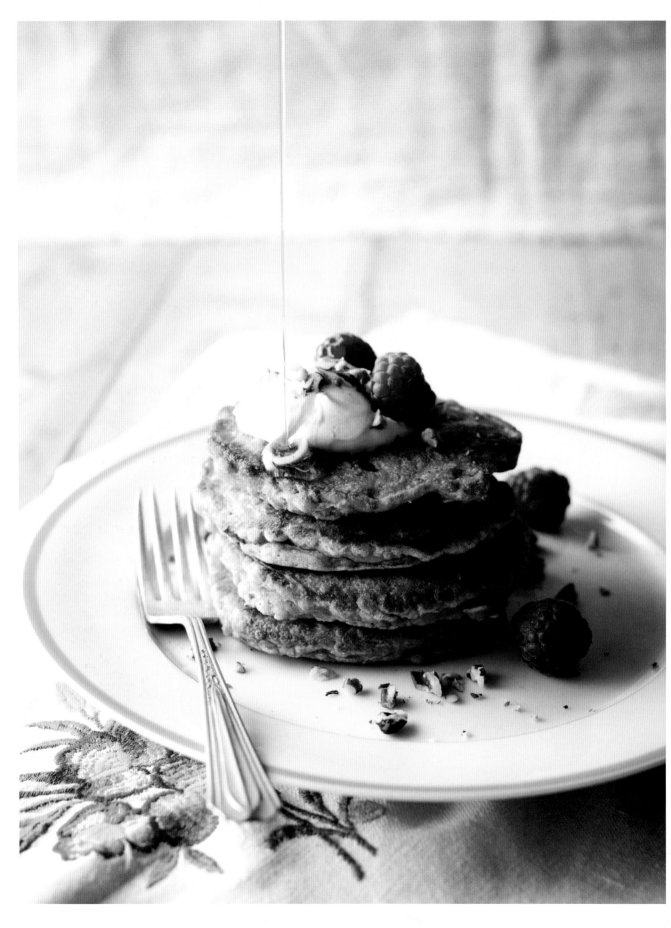

Oaty Pecan Pancakes

These indulgent wholemeal pancakes are a bit like drop scones, but have extra substance and flavour thanks to the oats and pecans. Delicious eaten straight from the pan or once cooled, popped in the toaster.

Makes 10-12

120g gluten-free rolled oats
120g buckwheat flour
1 tsp ground cinnamon
1 tsp baking powder
1 pinch salt
1 egg
2 tsp vanilla essence
1 tbsp maple syrup
270ml almond milk (or any
  milk of your choice)
40g pecan nuts, chopped
1 tbsp coconut oil

• DAIRY-FREE
• GLUTEN-FREE

1. Mix the oats, flour, cinnamon, baking powder and salt in a bowl.

2. In a separate bowl, whisk the egg, then pour in the vanilla essence, maple syrup and milk and stir well. Make a well in the centre of the dry ingredients, pour in the wet ingredients and gradually stir them in, followed by the nuts. The mixture should be thick but pourable. Allow it to rest for about 15 minutes.

3. Melt half the coconut oil in a frying pan over a medium heat. Drop blobs of the mixture into the pan, using 1-2 tablespoonfuls for each pancake. Repeat, leaving space around each one, and cook them for 2-3 minutes until they're golden brown and holes appear on the surface.

4. Flip them over carefully with a spatula and cook them for 1-2 minutes on the other side. Repeat with the remaining mixture.

5. They taste great served with 1 tbsp Greek-style yoghurt (add 75 cals), 1 tsp honey (add 20 cals) and some berries or half a sliced banana (add 50 cals).

130 CALORIES

Puddings

Even a healthy microbiome can enjoy an occasional good pud... though best after a meal rather than as a snack, and avoided in Phase 1.

Kefir and Berry Fool

This fool is a great way to jazz up kefir milk, and takes minutes to assemble.

Serves 2
200ml kefir
1½ tsp xanthum gum
1 tsp vanilla essence
100g Strawberry Chia 'Jam'
  (see below)
100g raspberries
50g blueberries

•GLUTEN-FREE

1. Whisk together the kefir, xanthum gum and vanilla essence.

2. Layer the mixture in 2 glasses with the jam and berries.

Tip: drizzle a little maple syrup on top if you have a sweet tooth.

140 CALORIES

Strawberry Chia 'Jam'

Makes about 10 tbsp
25g soft pitted dates, diced
  (or 1-2 tbsp date syrup)
1 tbsp balsamic vinegar
250g ripe strawberries,
  hulled and chopped
1 tbsp chia seeds

You will also need:
250ml jam jar with lid

•DAIRY-FREE
•GLUTEN-FREE

1. In a medium-sized pan, gently heat the dates with 2 tbsp water and the vinegar, stirring and pressing them with a spoon, to form a slightly lumpy paste.

2. Add the strawberries and continue to cook on a low heat for 4-5 minutes, then remove the pan from the heat, add the chia seeds and mash them into the softened strawberries with a spoon or masher.

3. Spoon the mixture into a small jar, and once it's cool put the lid on. The 'jam' can be stored in the fridge for up to a week.

20 CALORIES PER TBSP

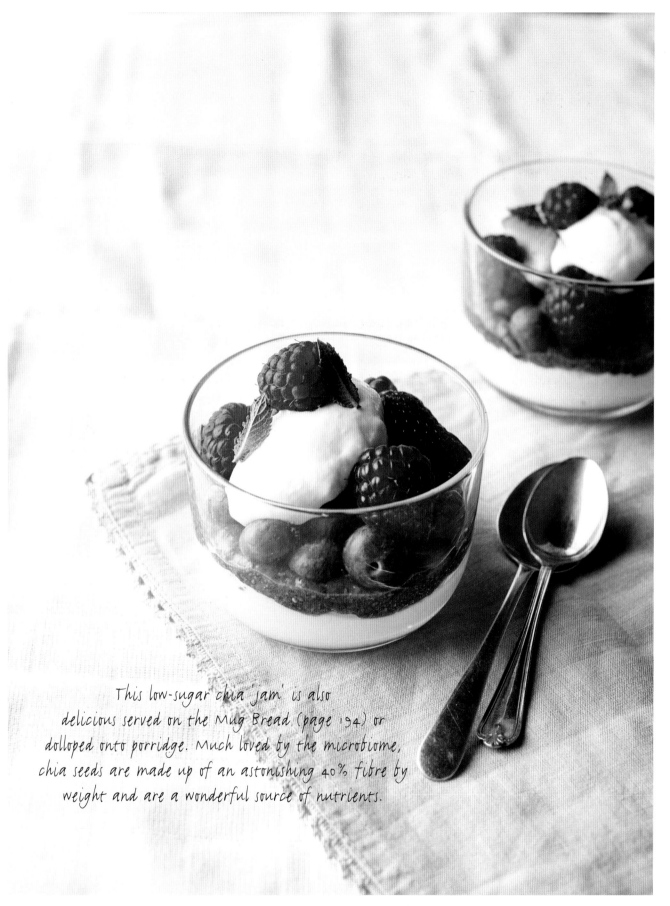

This low-sugar chia 'jam' is also
delicious served on the Mug Bread (page 194) or
dolloped onto porridge. Much loved by the microbiome,
chia seeds are made up of an astonishing 40% fibre by
weight and are a wonderful source of nutrients.

Purple Sweet Potato and Blackberry Pie

Purple sweet potato and blackberries are both top-of-the-range sources of soluble and insoluble fibre, and together they make a perfect pudding. The oil added here reduces the GI while increasing the absorption of nutrients, such as antioxidant carotenes. Blackberries bring a burst of fruity flavour along with a shot of vitamin C. If you can't find purple sweet potatoes, orange work well, too.

Serves 8

For the crust:

80g butter or coconut oil
20g light muscovado sugar
120g ground almonds
100g ground flaxseeds
30g desiccated coconut
¼ tsp Maldon sea salt

For the filling:

250g purple (or orange)
　sweet potatoes, peeled
　and diced
150g blackberries
30g ground flaxseeds
60g coconut oil
40g pitted dates, diced
1 tsp vanilla essence
1 tsp ground cinnamon
1 egg
100g blackberries or
　raspberries to serve

• DAIRY-FREE
• GLUTEN-FREE
• GOOD FOR PHASE 1

1. Preheat the oven to 160°C/140°C fan/gas mark 3. Lightly grease a 20cm loose-bottomed flan tin.

2. Melt the butter or coconut oil in a medium-sized pan. Add the sugar, and stir until it has dissolved. Remove the pan from the heat and stir in the remaining crust ingredients. Press the mixture into the bottom and sides of the prepared tin. Bake it in the middle of the oven for 20-25 minutes. The crust needs to be slightly golden and dry to the touch.

3. Meanwhile, steam the sweet potatoes for 15-20 minutes, until they're soft. Then blend them thoroughly with the other filling ingredients in a food processor. Pour the mixture into the pie crust and spread it evenly.

4. Bake the pie in the middle of the oven for 15-20 minutes, until it is set in the middle and starting to turn golden brown. Allow it to cool, then scatter the blackberries or raspberries on top before serving. Tastes great with a dollop of the Kefir Ginger Ice Cream (page 213).

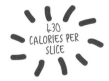

430 CALORIES PER SLICE

Dark Chocolate Avocado Mousse with Cashew Cream

A dark chocolate mousse to be eaten with a teaspoon and savoured – perfect at the end of a meal. Thanks to Dara Sutin for her recipe for the delicious low-carb Cardamom Cashew Cream to drizzle over the top.

Serves 6

160ml can coconut cream
40g cocoa powder
8 soft pitted dates, chopped
   (or 2-3 tbsp maple syrup
   or honey)
2 ripe avocados, flesh
   scooped out
1 tbsp coconut oil
1 tsp vanilla essence
1 ½ tbsp balsamic vinegar
150g raspberries

• DAIRY-FREE
• GLUTEN-FREE
• GOOD FOR PHASE 1

1. In a small saucepan, heat the coconut cream with the cocoa powder and the dates. Bring it to a simmer and stir for 1-2 minutes, then set it aside to cool for 5 minutes or so.

2. Pour the mixture, along with all the other ingredients, except the raspberries, into a food processor and blitz to form a smooth, creamy paste.

3. Divide the mixture between 6 small teacups, pots or glasses. Scatter the raspberries (or other berries or chopped ripe pear) over the top. Cool the mousse in the fridge before serving.

270 CALORIES

For the Cardamom Cashew Cream

A luxurious, versatile alternative to dairy cream.

Makes 6 portions

200g cashews, soaked in
   water for 2 hours
1 tsp vanilla essence
Tiny pinch of salt
1 tbsp maple syrup
Seeds from 2
   cardamom pods
100-150ml cold water

1. Drain the cashews, place them in a food processor with the vanilla, salt, maple syrup and cardamom seeds and pulse a couple of times.

2. Gradually add the water, blending until you have a smooth, creamy consistency.

3. Store any leftover Cashew Cream in an airtight container in the fridge for up to 3 days.

210 CALORIES

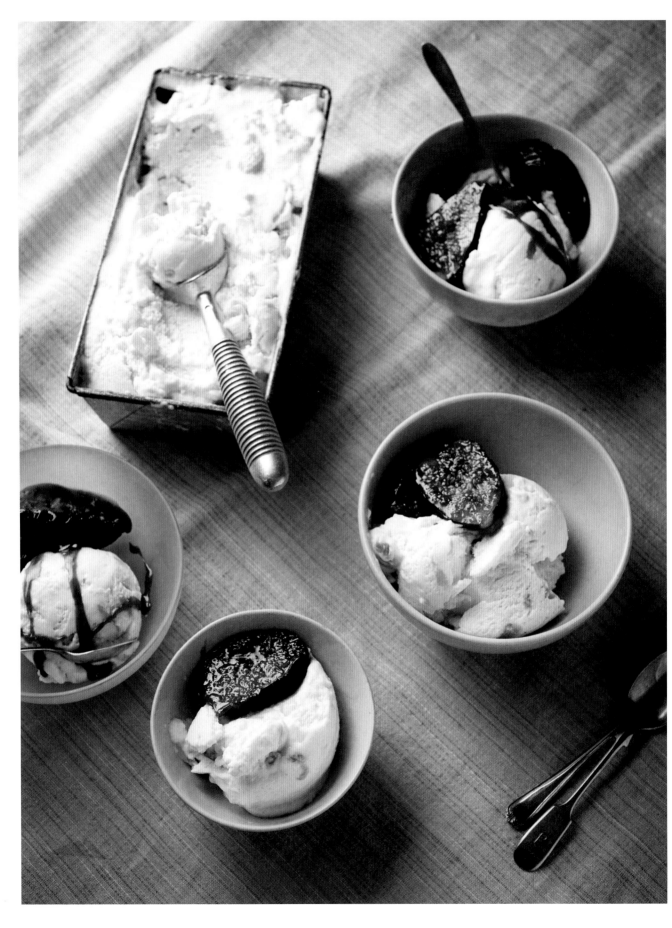

Kefir Ginger Ice Cream

Made with live kefir cultures, which contain a far richer variety of healthy bacteria than live yoghurt. Delicious served with baked or stewed fruits, such as figs, apple or rhubarb.

Serves 4
350ml kefir
160ml can coconut cream
2 tsp xanthum gum
3 pieces of stem ginger,
   finely diced

• GLUTEN-FREE

1. Place the kefir, coconut cream and xanthum gum in a bowl and whisk them together until smooth. Stir in the ginger, then pour the mixture into a freezer-proof container.

2. Place it in the freezer, removing it every half-hour for 2-3 hours and whisking it to break up the ice crystals.

3. Remove it from the freezer about 20-30 minutes before serving to allow it to soften.

Tip: alternatively, use an ice-cream maker!

200 CALORIES

Red Rice Pudding

An ideal way to use up leftover rice that has already been converted to resistant starch by being cooled for 12 hours. Creamy, nutty and exotic.

Serves 4
400g precooked red and
   brown rice
400ml can coconut milk
¾ tsp ground cinnamon
½ tsp ground nutmeg
Seeds from 8-10
   cardamom pods
1 tsp vanilla essence
1½ tbsp maple syrup
Pinch of salt

• DAIRY-FREE

• GLUTEN-FREE

• GOOD FOR PHASE 1

1. Place all in the ingredients in a medium-sized saucepan and bring it to a simmer.

2. Continue to simmer, stirring occasionally, for 15 minutes, until the consistency is loose and creamy.

Note: to cook the rice in advance, place 75g red rice and 75g brown rice in a pan of simmering water for 15-18 minutes, or until tender. Drain, refresh with cold water, then drain again. Store it in the fridge for 12 hours.

330 CALORIES

MEAL PLANNERS

Phase 1

The **Phase 1** menu plans are a guide to help ensure you have a varied diet with a good balance of nutrients during these few weeks when you are restricting ingredients. Adjust the plan to your tastes. Skip foods that you know don't suit you. This phase is mainly gluten-free and dairy-free; it is also low in pulses (though vegetarians should reintroduce these after 2 weeks to maintain their protein intake).

Before you start Phase 1, we recommend you record your baseline symptoms and eating habits for at least 3 days on the Daily Food and Symptoms Diary (download from cleverguts.com).

We have generally included more substantial meals in the 'supper' category on the basis that many people have more time available in the evening; however, the earlier in the day that you eat your main meal, the better for weight loss, and your metabolism and microbiome. We also propose a few days when you might have a generous breakfast and skip lunch, to give your gut a brief recovery and repair period. In general, try to fast for at least 12 hours overnight.

We have not offered a menu plan for **Phase 2** (for more information on this go to page 27), since all the recipes in this book are suitable for this phase. In Phase 2, we particularly encourage you to include more prebiotic veg, such as Jerusalem artichokes and chicory; and more probiotic, fermented foods such as kefir milk and Red Cabbage Sauerkraut (see chapter 6). Try to increase your consumption of multicoloured vegetables and fruit and include some grains. In this phase, you get to enjoy occasional treats, too (see chapter 7).

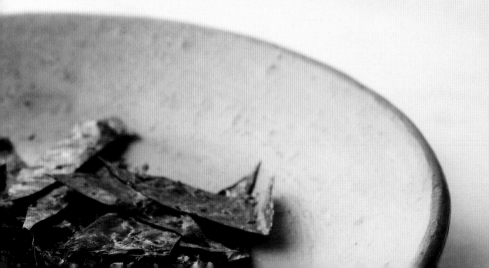

	Breakfast	Lunch	Dinner
Monday	Creamy Scrambled Eggs with smoked salmon (pg 37)	Citrus salad (pg 55) with Turmeric Buttermilk dressing (pg 119)	Baked Coconut Chicken Curry (pg 126) with 2 tbsp Red Rice with Resistant Starch (pg 176) and steamed leafy greens
Tuesday	Blueberry Chia Pot with 1 tbsp of berries (pg 45)	Green Gazpacho Soup with Seaweed (pg 63)	Prosciutto Wrapped Pork Loin (pg 149) with Creamy Nutmeg Spinach (pg 160)
Wednesday	Turmeric and Coconut Spiced Omelette with Seaweed (pg 38)	Smoked Salmon Ceviche (pg 84) with Thai Seaweed Crackers (pg 79)	Bitter Leaf and Pine Nut Salad (pg 56) with Cider Vinegar Dressing (pg 117), followed by Michael's Mussels (pg 98)
Thursday	Coconut Porridge with Pecans and Pear (pg 42)	Crab Spaghetti with Seaweed (pg 101)	Steak with Guacamole and Blistered Tomatoes (pg 153)
Friday	Sour Cream and Seaweed Muffin (pg 83)	Chinese Noodle Jar (pg 70)	Baked Salmon with Seaweed Pesto (pg 132) and Beets Roasted (pg 170)
Saturday	Bircher Muesli (pg 45)	Skip lunch	Beef and Orange Stew (pg 150) with Pan-Fried Courgetti Spaghetti (pg 177)
Sunday	Creamy Scrambled Eggs with Avocado (pg 37)	Mackerel with Quinoa Tabbouleh (pg 106)	Easy Chicken Tagine (pg 127) and Red Rice with Resistant Starch (pg 176)

	Breakfast	Lunch	Dinner
Monday	Creamy Scrambled Eggs with Smoked Salmon (pg 37)	Phyto Salad (pg 66)	Vegetable and Paneer Curry (pg 145) with 1 tbsp Greek Yoghurt and 2 tbsp cooked, cooled and reheated brown rice
Tuesday	Coconut Porridge with berries (pg 42)	Turkey and Mushroom Bolognese (pg 131) with Pan-fried Courgetti Spaghetti (pg 177)	Turmeric Coronation Chicken (pg 111), Cauli Rice and Coriander (pg 174) and steamed leafy veg
Wednesday	Avocado with Smoked Salmon (pg 46)	Terra Mare Squid Salad (pg 88) with 2 tbsp quinoa	Marinated Tofu Stir-fry with GF Noodles (pg 144)
Thursday	Speedy Kippers with Blistered Tomatoes (pg 46)	Past with Pistachio Pesto (pg 99) with Citrus Salad (page 55) or steamed veg	Thai Prawns with Coconut Milk (pg 141) with 2 tbsp cooked, cooled and reheated brown rice
Friday	Pineapple Smoothie (pg 51)	Tuna and Veg Stir-fry with Seaweed (pg 109)	Michael's' Mussels (pg 98) with 2 slices of Mug Bread (pg 194)
Saturday	Breakfast Fry-up with Green Banana (pg 41)	Healing Chicken Bone Broth (pg 59)	Lazy Lemon and Lime Chicken (pg 130) and Creamy Nutmeg Spinach (pg 56)
Sunday	Creamy Scrambled Eggs with Fried Mushrooms (pg 37)	Skip lunch	Seafood with Seaweed Risotto (pg 139) with Garlic Stir-fried Greens (pg 161)

	Breakfast	Lunch	Dinner
Monday	Dr Tim's Healthy Gut Smoothie (pg 50)	Citrus Salad (pg 55) with Avocado and Lime Salsa (pg 75)	Veira's Coriander Chicken (pg 128) with Spinach Dahl (pg 112) and 2 tbsp quinoa
Tuesday	Creamy Scrambled Eggs with leafy veg and Parmesan (pg 37)	Smoked Salmon Ceviche with a leafy green salad (pg 84)	Mackerel with Spiced Coconut (pg 133) and Beets Roasted (pg 177) and steamed leafy greens
Wednesday	Kale and Tofu Scramble (pg 93)	Warm Red Rice Salad with Courgette (pg 90)	Sea Bass with Seaweed Salsa Verde (pg 135) and Roasted Butternut Squash (pg 172)
Thursday	Clever Guts Green Smoothie (pg 48)	Pink Celeriac and Beetroot soup (pg 64) with Flaxseed Crackers (pg 78)	Black Bean Beet Burgers (pg 147) with Quick Garlic Fried Greens (pg 161) and 2 tbsp quinoa
Friday	Turmeric and Coconut Spiced Omelette with Seaweed (pg 38)	Crab Spaghetti with Seaweed (pg 101) with steamed green and coloured veg	Bitter Leaf and Pine Nut Salad (pg 56) with Cider Vinegar Dressing (pg 117) followed by Mackerel with Quinoa Tabbouleh (pg 106)
Saturday	Coconut Porridge with Pecans and Pears (pg 42)	Poor Man's Potatoes with Anchovies (pg 102)	Easy Chicken Tagine (pg 127) with Roasted Butternut Squash (pg 172)
Sunday	Creamy Scrambled Eggs (pg 37) with Slow Roast Tomatoes (pg 172)	Green Banana and Peppers Stir-fry (pg 163)	A bitter leaf salad (page 55-6) followed by Sweet Potato, Kale and Cod Fishcakes (pg 136) and Aubergine Chips (pg 175)

	Breakfast	Lunch	Dinner
Monday	Blueberry Chia Pot (pg 45)	Phyto Salad Bowl (pg 66)	Turmeric Coronation Chicken (pg 111) with Red Rice with Resistant Starch (pg 176) and steamed veg
Tuesday	Clever Guts Green Smoothie (pg 48)	Smoked Mackerel and Kale Kedgeree (pg 47) with Slow Roast Tomatoes (pg 172)	Aubergine Parmigiana (pg 96) with steamed coloured and dark leafy greens
Wednesday	Speedy Kippers (pg 46) with Creamy Scrambled Eggs (pg 37)	Bitter Leaves and Toasted Pine Nut Salad (pg 56) with Lime Dressing (pg 116)	Marinated Tofu Stir Fry with Noodles (pg 144)
Thursday	Yoghurt with Chia Jam and Toasted Pistachios (pg 35)	Roasted Mediterranean Vegetables, Pearl Barley and Eggs (pg 105)	Sausage and Mediterranean Veg Bake (pg 154) with 2 tbsp brown rice or quinoa
Friday	Bircher Muesli made with non-dairy milk (pg 45)	Pistachio Pesto (pg 99) with Garlic Fried Greens (pg 161)	Squid Provencal (pg 142) with 2 tbsp brown rice or quinoa
Saturday	Breakfast Fry-up with Green Bananas (pg 41)	Skip lunch	Turkey and Mushroom Bolognese (pg 131) with Pan-Fried Courgetti Spaghetti (pg 177)
Sunday	Pineapple Smoothie (pg 51)	Spicy Lentil and Tomato Soup (pg 62) with Flaxseed Crackers (pg 78)	Beef and Orange Stew (pg 150) with Cauliflower Baked with Lemon and Almonds (pg 95) and steamed greens

Planner for 5:2 Days (800 calories a day)

Feel free to swap the lunch and supper menus around. Steamed leafy veg or crudités add only a few extra calories and add fibre so you can top up with these. If skipping a meal is proving difficult, have some hot Miso Seaweed Soup or Gut-Soothing Vegetable Bouillon to tide you over. For more on how Intermittent Fasting can help heal your gut, see page 18.

Breakfast	Lunch	Dinner	Cals
Creamy Scrambled Eggs with Smoked Salmon (280, pg 37)	Skip lunch	Easy Chicken Tagine with Preserved Lemons (470, pg 127) Red Rice with Resistant Starch (90, pg 176)	840
Turmeric and Coconut Spiced Omelette with Seaweed (270, pg 38)	Pink Celeriac and Beetroot Soup (210, pg 64)	Mackerel and Quinoa Tabbouleh (410, pg 106)	890
Yoghurt with Chia Jam and Pistachios (230, pg 35)	Chargrilled Red Pepper Dip (160, pg 73) with Cucumber Crudités	Steak with Guacamole and Blistered Tomatoes (470, pg 153)	860
Avocado with Smoked Salmon (280, pg 46)	Skip lunch	Lazy Lemon and Lime Baked Chicken (560, pg 130) with steamed greens	840
Creamy Scrambled Eggs with Smoked Salmon (280, pg 37)	Tuna and Veg Stir-fry with Seaweed (270, pg 109)	Roasted Butternut Squash (240, pg 172) and Scorched Radicchio (10, pg 160)	800
Pineapple Smoothie (460, pg 51)	Quick Miso Soup (20, pg 61) with 1 Thai Seaweed Cracker (60, pg 79)	Bitter Leaves and Toasted Pine Nut Salad (260, pg 56)	800
Creamy Scrambled Eggs (190, pg 37)	Garlic Fried Greens (290, pg 161)	Quorn and Parsnip Pie (410, pg 148)	890
Sour Cream and Seaweed Muffin (200, pg 83)	2 x Spinach and Ricotta Blini (240, pg 80) with half serving of Smoked Mackerel Pàté (80, pg 75)	Brazilian-Style Crab (370, pg 110) with steamed green vegetables	890
Creamy Scrambled Eggs (190, pg 37)	Citrus Salad (100, pg 55) with Turmeric Buttermilk Dressing (70, pg 119)	Prosciutto Wrapped Pork (420, pg 149) Red Rice with RS (90, pg 176)	870
Dr Tim's Healthy Gut Smoothie (520, pg 50)	Skip lunch	Sea Bass with Seaweed Salsa Verde (380, pg 135) and steamed green veg	900
1 Spinach and Ricotta Blini (120, pg 80) with slice of smoked salmon (90)	Quick Miso Soup (20, pg 61), Flaxseed Cracker (80, pg 78)	Sausage and Mediterranean Bake (510, pg 154)	820
Creamy Scrambled Eggs 190, pg 37)	Spicy Lentil and Tomato Soup (160, pg 62)	Sweet Potato, Kale and Cod Fishcakes (340, pg 136) Citrus Salad (100, pg 55) with Lemony Buttermilk Dressing (70, pg 118)	860
1 Apricot and Pistachio Bar (220, pg 201)	Smoked Mackerel Pàté with (160, pg 75) and 2 Flaxseed Crackers (160, pg 78)	Green Beans and Edamame with Anchovies (240, pg 87)	780
Clever Guts Smoothie (450, pg 48)	Skip lunch	Smoked Salmon Ceviche (450, pg 84)	900
1 Oaty Pecan Pancake (130, pg 207)	Chinese Noodle Jar (300, pg 70)	Tofu Stir-Fry with Noodles (410, pg 144)	840

Acknowledgements

I am hugely appreciative to Michael for involving me in the exciting new world of gut health and for testing some strange concoctions with good humour and wise advice. Likewise, thanks to all four children, Alex, Jack, Dan and Kate, for their encouragement and honest feedback (!). And particularly for the invaluable insights from one who turned out to be gluten-intolerant during the writing of the book and remains happily gluten-free.

Special thanks to Rebecca Nicolson and the rest of the talented team at Short Books, editor Aurea Carpenter for her vision, turn of phrase and excellent guidance, Paul Bougourd, and Andrew Smith for his design.

A big thank you to consultant nutritionist Joy Skipper for testing, advising, contributing delicious recipes and ensuring all is nutritionally sound, and also to Sue Camp for excellent advice and recipe analysis.

The wonderful, luscious images were created by photographer Joe Sarah and food stylist Dara Sutin.

Thanks also to friends and family who have patiently answered endless questions about traditional cooking, recipes and fermentation, including my niece Emily, an expert in Japanese food, mother-in-law Joan, step-mother Wendy, brother Aidan, sister-in-laws Nikki and Sylvia, and great friend, cook and ferment soulmate, Caroline Barton. Also to my mother, a superb and adventurous cook, who celebrated food, taught us to cook and would have loved to have been involved.

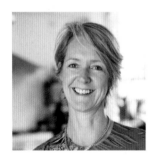

Dr. Clare Bailey is a general practitioner doing diet research with Oxford University. She is the author of *The 8-Week Blood Sugar Diet Cookbook*, and is married to Dr. Michael Mosley, author of *The Clever Gut Diet*, *The Fast Diet*, and *The 8 Week Blood Sugar Diet*. She is also founder of Parenting Matters, an organisation that helps parents become more confident through courses and one to one consultations.

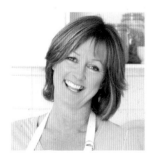

Joy Skipper is a qualified nutritionist who has worked in the food industry for over twenty years, writing cookbooks and advising clients on healthy diet and lifestyle.

Index

5:2 diet 11, 19, 217

abdominal fat 22
activity 22
Akkermansia 18, 201
allergic diseases 6, 23
almonds
   aubergines chips 175
   cauliflower baked with lemon
     and almonds 95
   mug bread 194
amino acids 106
anchovies
   anchovy and rosemary dressing
     116
   green beans and edamame with
     anchovies 87
   poor man's potatoes and
     anchovies 102
   prawns with pasta and seaweed
     141
   salsa verde with seaweed 117
antibiotics 6
antioxidants 14, 94
appetite 20
apple cider vinegar
   beef and orange stew with
     mushrooms 150
   bitter leaves and toasted pine
     nut salad 56
   chicken bone broth 59
   cider vinegar tipple 56
   dressing 117
   green gazpacho with seaweed
     63
   Japanese-style quick pickled
     veg 167
   nutrition 17, 56
   Quorn and parsnip cottage
     pie 148
   salsa verde with seaweed 117
apricots
   apricot and pistachio bars 201
   chicken tagine with preserved
     lemons 127
   turmeric coronation chicken
     111
   healthy homemade granola 34
   pistachio and olive oil cake
     204
asparagus
   broccoli and asparagus with
     buttermilk dressing 90
   citrus, fennel and asparagus
     salad 55
aubergines 24
   aubergine parmigiana 96
   chips 175
   chocolate aubergine cake 202
   Mediterranean roasted veg,

     pearl barley and eggs 105
   smoky with cannellini beans
     164
   vegetable and paneer curry
     145
avocado
   avocado and lime salsa 75
   avocado and smoked salmon
     46
   chocolate avocado mousse with
     cashew cream 211
   clever guts green smoothie 48
   Dr Tim's smoothie 50
   phyto salad lunchbox 69
   smoked salmon ceviche 84
   steak with guacamole and
     blistered tomatoes 153

bacon, breakfast fry-up with
   green bananas 41
bananas
   breakfast fry-up with green
     bananas 41
   green banana and pepper stir-
     fry 163
   bean sprouts, marinated tofu
     with noodles 144
beans
   black bean beet burgers 147
   smoky aubergine with
     cannellini beans 164
beef
   beef and orange stew with
     mushrooms 150
   steak with guacamole and
     blistered tomatoes 153
beetroot
   beetroot and chilli cream
     cheese spread 77
   beetroot and yoghurt dip 72
   beets roasted in their skins
     170
   black bean beet burgers 147
   celeriac and beetroot soup 64
   mackerel with quinoa
     tabbouleh 106
berries
   kefir and berry fool 208
   yoghurt with chia jam and
     toasted pistachios 35
bhajis, onion and courgette 162
bircher muesli with kefir 45
bitter leaves and toasted pine nut
   salad 56
black bean beet burgers 147
blackberries, purple sweet potato
   and blackberry pie 210
blinis, spinach and ricotta 80
blood orange salad with toasted
   coriander 55

blood sugar 18, 19, 20, 59
blue cheese butter 121
blueberries
   blueberry chia pots 45
   clever guts green smoothie 48
   Dr Tim's smoothie 50
bouillon, vegetable 60
Brazilian-style crab 110
breads
   mug bread 194
   no-knead sourdough 198–9
   seeded soda bread 196
   wholewheat flatbread 195
breakfast 20
   breakfast fry-up with green
     bananas 41
broccoli
   and asparagus with buttermilk
     dressing 90
   mac 'n' cheese, low-carb 92
   marinated tofu with noodles
     144
   Thai prawns with coconut milk
     and seaweed 138
   toasted slaw with halloumi and
     lemony buttermilk dressing
     89
broths, chicken bone broth 59
buttermilk
   lemony buttermilk dressing
     118
   sour cream and seaweed
     muffins 83
   toasted slaw with halloumi and
     lemony buttermilk dressing
     89
   turmeric buttermilk dressing
     119
butternut squash
   Mediterranean roasted veg,
     pearl barley and eggs 105
   pasta with pistachio pesto 99
   Quorn and parsnip cottage
     pie 148
   roasted 172
   turkey and mushroom
     bolognese 131
butters, flavoured 121

cabbage
   breakfast fry-up with green
     bananas 41
   mushroom omelette with red
     sauerkraut 38
   red cabbage sauerkraut 185
   toasted slaw with halloumi and
     lemony buttermilk dressing
     89
   tuna and veg stir-fry with
     seaweed 109

warm red rice salad with courgettes 90
cakes
  chocolate and aubergine 202
  exotic carrot 205
  pistachio and olive oil 204
calorie intake 11
cannellini beans, with smoky aubergine 164
carbohydrates, starchy 10
cardamom cashew cream 211
carotenoids 67
carrots
  beef and orange stew with mushrooms 150
  carrot cake 205
  chicken bone broth 59
  mackerel with quinoa tabbouleh 106
  roasted purple with tarragon 171
  turkey and mushroom bolognese 131
  vegetable bouillon 60
cashews
  bircher muesli with kefir 45
  cardamom cashew cream 211
  chickpea, coconut and cashew curry 107
  Chinese noodle jar 70
  chocolate avocado mousse with cashew cream 211
  creamy pineapple smoothie 51
  marinated tofu with noodles 144
cauliflower
  baked with lemon and almonds 95
  broccoli and asparagus with buttermilk dressing 90
  mac 'n' cheese, low-carb 92
  rice with coriander 174
  smoked mackerel and kale kedgeree 47
  vegetable and paneer curry 145
celeriac
  celeriac and beetroot soup 64
  Quorn and parsnip cottage pie 148
celery
  beef and orange stew with mushrooms 150
  chicken bone broth 59
  chickpea, coconut and cashew curry 107
  clever guts green smoothie 48
  coriander chicken with yoghurt and fennel 128
  prawns with pasta and seaweed 141
  tuna and veg stir-fry with seaweed 109
  vegetable bouillon 60

ceviche, smoked salmon 84
cheese
  aubergine parmigiana 96
  black bean beet burgers 147
  blue cheese butter 121
  broccoli and asparagus with buttermilk dressing 90
  mac 'n' cheese, low-carb 92
  Mediterranean roasted veg, pearl barley and eggs 105
  pasta with pistachio pesto 99
  scrambled eggs with leafy veg and Parmesan 37
  sour cream and seaweed muffins 83
  spinach dahl 112
  toasted slaw with halloumi and lemony buttermilk dressing 89
  vegetable and paneer curry 145
  warm lentil salad 87
chia seeds
  blueberry chia pots 45
  flaxseed crackers 78
  nutrition 209
  seeded soda bread 196
  strawberry chia 'jam' 208
  yoghurt with chia jam and toasted pistachios 35
chicken
  coconut chicken curry, baked 126
  coriander chicken with yoghurt and fennel 128
  turmeric coronation chicken 111
  lemon and lime baked chicken 130
  tagine with preserved lemons 127
chicken bone broth 59
chickpeas
  chickpea, coconut and cashew curry 107
  lemon and coriander hummus with seaweed 74
Chinese noodle jar 70
chocolate and walnut bites 202
chocolate aubergine cake 202
chocolate avocado mousse with cashew cream 211
citrus, fennel and asparagus salad 55
Clever Guts diet
  phase one 25, 214–16
  phase two 27
coconut, dry sambal 120
coconut cream
  chocolate avocado mousse with cashew cream 211
  kefir ginger ice cream 213
coconut milk
  baked coconut chicken curry

126
  blueberry chia pots 45
  Brazilian-style crab 110
  chickpea, coconut and cashew curry 107
  coconut porridge with pecans and pear 42
  red rice pudding 213
  spinach dahl 112
  Thai prawns with coconut milk and seaweed 138
cod, sweet potato, kale and cod fishcakes 136
coeliac disease 23
coriander chicken with yoghurt and fennel 128
coronation chicken with turmeric 111
cortisol 22
cottage pie, Quorn and parsnip 148
courgettes
  baked salmon with seaweed pesto 132
  crab spaghetti with seaweed 101
  Mediterranean roasted veg, pearl barley and eggs 105
  onion and courgette bhajis 162
  pan-fried courgetti spaghetti 177
  pasta with pistachio pesto 99
  pickled with mustard seeds 188
  sausage and Mediterranean veg tray bake 154
  turkey and mushroom bolognese 131
  warm red rice salad with courgettes 90
crab
  Brazilian-style 110
  crab spaghetti with seaweed 101
crackers
  flaxseed 78
  Thai-flavoured seaweed 79
cranberries
  bircher muesli with kefir 45
  healthy homemade granola 34
cream cheese spreads 77
cruciferous vegetables 94
curcumin 17, 111
curries
  baked coconut chicken 126
  chickpea, coconut and cashew curry 107
  coconut chicken curry, baked 126
  spinach dahl 112
  vegetable and paneer curry 145

dahl, spinach 112

dairy foods 12–13, 27, 77
dates
  apricot and pistachio bars 201
  chocolate and walnut bites 202
  chocolate avocado mousse with
    cashew cream 211
  exotic carrot cake 205
  healthy homemade granola 34
  purple sweet potato and
    blackberry pie 210
  strawberry chia 'jam' 208
diabetes type 2 6, 10, 19, 66
diary keeping 24, 27
digestive enzyme production 11
dips
  beetroot and yoghurt 72
  chargrilled red pepper 73
dressings
  anchovy and rosemary 116
  apple cider vinegar 117
  kefir mustard 119
  lemony buttermilk 118
  lime 116
  pesto kefir 119
  salsa verde with seaweed 117
  turmeric buttermilk 119
drinks 19
  clever guts green smoothie 48
  creamy pineapple smoothie 51
  Dr Tim's smoothie 50
kombucha 180–2
  turmeric tea 21

edamame beans
  Chinese noodle jar 70
  green beans and edamame with
    anchovies 87
  pea and edamame mash 162
  smoked salmon ceviche 84
eggs
  Mediterranean roasted veg,
    pearl barley and eggs 105
  mushroom omelette with red
    sauerkraut 38
  nutrition 17
  scrambled 37
  smoked mackerel and kale
    kedgeree 47
  spinach and ricotta blinis 80
  turmeric spiced omelette with
    seaweed 38
exclusion diets 13
exercise 22

fats 12, 17
fennel
  citrus, fennel and asparagus
    salad 55
  coriander chicken with yoghurt
    and fennel 128
  prawns with pasta and seaweed
    141
  prosciutto-wrapped pork loin
    149

fermented foods 8, 14, 17
fibre 13–14
fish
  anchovy and rosemary dressing
    116
  avocado and smoked salmon
    46
  baked salmon with seaweed
    pesto 132
  green beans and edamame with
    anchovies 87
  kippers 46
  mackerel fillets with spiced
    coconut 133
  mackerel with quinoa
    tabbouleh 106
  nutrition 12, 17, 46
  phyto salad lunchbox 69
  poor man's potatoes and
    anchovies 102
  sea bass with seaweed salsa
    verde 135
  smoked mackerel and kale
    kedgeree 47
  smoked mackerel pâté 75
  smoked salmon ceviche 84
  smoked salmon cream cheese
    spread 77
  sweet potato, kale and cod
    fishcakes 136
  tuna and veg stir-fry with
    seaweed 109
flavonoids 67
flaxseed crackers 78
flour 13
FODMAPs 24
food allergies 23
food intolerances 6, 12, 23, 25
food labels 10
fructooligosacharides 14
fruit, variety 14, 17

garlic and parsley butter 121
gazpacho, green with seaweed
  63
gluten 13, 27
Glycaemic Index (GI) 10
grains 13
granola
  healthy homemade 34
    with yoghurt and pear 32
  green beans and edamame with
    anchovies 87
greens, quick garlic-fried 161
gut lining 18, 201

halloumi, toasted slaw with
halloumi and lemony buttermilk
  dressing 89
herb butter 121
horseradish cream cheese spread
  77
hummus, lemon and coriander
  with seaweed 74

IBS 14, 23, 24
ice cream, kefir ginger 213
immune system 22
inflammation 10, 24
ingredient planning 28–9
insulin 12
intermittent fasting (IF) 18 see
  also 5:2 diet
inulin 14, 20

Japanese-style quick pickled veg
  167
Jerusalem artichokes, roasted
  171

kale
  breakfast fry-up with green
    bananas 41
  clever guts green smoothie 48
  kale and tofu scramble 93
  smoked mackerel and kale
    kedgeree 47
  sweet potato, kale and cod
    fishcakes 136
kefir
  bircher muesli with kefir 45
  kefir and berry fool 208
  kefir ginger ice cream 213
kefir milk 190–1
kefir mustard dressing 119
  nutrition 54
  pesto kefir dressing 119
  seeded soda bread 196
kippers 46
kombucha 180–2

Lactobacillus 17, 189, 198
lactose intolerance 12–13
lamb, slow-roast shoulder 157
leaky gut syndrome 24
leeks
  chicken bone broth 59
  terra mare salad with marine
    Phukka 88
  vegetable bouillon 60
lemons
  cauliflower baked with lemon
    and almonds 95
  chicken tagine with preserved
    lemons 127
  lemon and coriander hummus
    with seaweed 74
  lemon and lime baked chicken
    130
  lemon and pepper butter 121
  lemony buttermilk dressing
    118
  preserved 184
  terra mare salad with marine
    Phukka 88
  warm red rice salad with
    courgettes 90
lentils
  lentil and tomato soup 62

Puy lentils with balsamic
   vinegar 169
spinach dahl 112
warm salad 87
limes
   avocado and lime salsa 75
   Brazilian-style crab 110
   chickpea, coconut and cashew
      curry 107
   dry coconut sambal 120
   lemon and lime baked chicken
      130
   lime dressing 116
   smoked salmon ceviche 84
   Thai prawns with coconut milk
      and seaweed 138

mac 'n' cheese, low-carb 92
mackerel
   mackerel fillets with spiced
      coconut 133
   mackerel with quinoa
      tabbouleh 106
   smoked mackerel and kale
      kedgeree 47
   smoked mackerel pâté 75
Marmite
   flaxseed crackers 78
   seaweed miso soup 61
meal plans 214–17
meat 12, 149, 157
medical checks 23
Mediterranean roasted veg,
   pearl barley and eggs 105
Mediterranean style food 10
metabolism 22
microbiome 6, 8, 22
milk, Dr Tim's smoothie 50
mindfulness 22
miso
   Chinese noodle jar 70
   seaweed miso soup 61
muffins, sour cream and seaweed
   83
mug bread 194
mushrooms
   beef and orange stew with
      mushrooms 150
   breakfast fry-up with green
      bananas 41
   lemon and lime baked chicken
      130
   mushroom omelette with red
      sauerkraut 38
   with scrambled eggs 37
   toasted slaw with halloumi and
      lemony buttermilk dressing
      89
   turkey and mushroom
      bolognese 131
mussels, Michael's 98
mustard butter 121
mustard seeds 94

nightshade vegetables 24
noodles
   Chinese noodle jar 70
   marinated tofu with noodles
      144
nuts
   apricot and pistachio bars 201
   aubergines chips 175
   bircher muesli with kefir 45
   blueberry chia pots 45
   cardamom cashew cream 211
   cauliflower baked with lemon
      and almonds 95
   chickpea, coconut and cashew
      curry 107
   Chinese noodle jar 70
   chocolate and walnut bites 202
   chocolate aubergine cake 202
   chocolate avocado mousse with
      cashew cream 211
   coconut porridge with pecans
      and pear 42
   exotic carrot cake 205
   marinated tofu with noodles
      144
   mug bread 194
   nut butter 123
   nutrition 17
   oaty pecan pancakes 207
   pasta with pistachio pesto 99
   pistachio and olive oil cake
      204
   yoghurt with chia jam and
      toasted pistachios 35

oats
   bircher muesli with kefir 45
   chocolate and walnut bites 202
   coconut porridge with pecans
      and pear 42
   healthy homemade granola 34
   oaty pecan pancakes 207
obesity 6
olive oil
   nutrition 17
   pistachio and olive oil cake
      204
omega 3 46
omelettes
   mushroom with red sauerkraut
      38
   turmeric spiced with seaweed
      38
onions
   avocado and lime salsa 75
   baked salmon with seaweed
      pesto 132
   blood orange salad with toasted
      coriander 55
   broccoli and asparagus with
      buttermilk dressing 90
   chicken bone broth 59
   chickpea, coconut and cashew
      curry 107

lemon and lime baked chicken
   130
onion and courgette bhajis 162
poor man's potatoes and
   anchovies 102
red cabbage sauerkraut 185
sausage and Mediterranean veg
   tray bake 154
smoked mackerel and kale
   kedgeree 47
spicy pickled 189
squid Provençal 142
tuna and veg stir-fry with
   seaweed 109
vegetable and paneer curry
   145
vegetable bouillon 60
warm lentil salad 87
oranges
   beef and orange stew with
      mushrooms 150
   blood orange salad with toasted
      coriander 55
   citrus, fennel and asparagus
      salad 55

pak choi, Dr Tim's smoothie 50
palette 11
pancetta, breakfast fry-up with
   green bananas 41
parsnips, Quorn and parsnip
   cottage pie 148
pasta
   crab spaghetti with seaweed
      101
   mac 'n' cheese, low-carb 92
   with pistachio pesto 99
   prawns with pasta and seaweed
      138
   Thai prawns with coconut milk
      and seaweed 141
pâté, smoked mackerel 75
pea and edamame mash 162
pearl barley, Mediterranean
   roasted veg, pearl barley
   and eggs 105
pears
   chocolate aubergine cake 202
   coconut porridge with pecans
      and pear 42
   yoghurt with granola and diced
      pear 32
pecans
   blueberry chia pots 45
   chocolate and walnut bites 202
   coconut porridge with pecans
      and pear 42
   oaty pecan pancakes 207
peppers (bell) 24
   baked coconut chicken curry
      126
   baked salmon with seaweed
      pesto 132

Brazilian-style crab 110
chargrilled red pepper dip 73
chicken tagine with preserved lemons 127
green banana and pepper stir-fry 163
marinated tofu with noodles 144
Mediterranean roasted veg, pearl barley and eggs 105
poor man's potatoes and anchovies 102
sausage and Mediterranean veg tray bake 154
smoked mackerel and kale kedgeree 47
squid Provençal 142
tuna and veg stir-fry with seaweed 109
vegetable and paneer curry 145
pesto kefir dressing 119
phyto salad 66–7
phyto salad lunchbox 69
phytonutrients 14, 67
pies, purple sweet potato and blackberry pie 210
pine nuts
    bitter leaves and toasted pine nut salad 56
    mackerel with quinoa tabbouleh 106
    warm red rice salad with courgettes 90
pineapple, creamy pineapple smoothie 51
pistachios
    apricot and pistachio bars 201
    pasta with pistachio pesto 99
    pistachio and olive oil cake 204
    yoghurt with chia jam and toasted pistachios 35
planning 19, 20, 214–17
polyphenols 14, 67
pork, prosciutto-wrapped pork loin 149
porridge, coconut porridge with pecans and pear 42
portion control 20
potatoes 24
    baked 11
    poor man's potatoes and anchovies 102
prawns
    nutrition 140
    with pasta and seaweed 138
    Thai prawns with coconut milk and seaweed 141
prebiotics 14, 27, 40
probiotics 8, 14, 27, 56
processed foods 10
prosciutto-wrapped pork loin 149

protein
    intake 12, 157
    variety 12
proteins, variety 8
Puy lentils with balsamic vinegar 169

quinoa
    black bean beet burgers 147
    lemon and lime baked chicken 130
    mackerel with quinoa tabbouleh 106
    phyto salad lunchbox 69
    terra mare salad with marine Phukka 88
Quorn and parsnip cottage pie 148

radicchio, scorched purple 160
red peppers see peppers (bell)
resistant starch 40, 41, 176
riboflavin 106
rice
    red rice pudding 213
    red rice with resistant starch 176
    seafood with seaweed risotto 139
    smoked mackerel and kale kedgeree 47
    warm red rice salad with courgettes 90
ricotta, spinach and ricotta blinis 80

salads
    bitter leaves and toasted pine nut 56
    blood orange with toasted coriander 55
    citrus, fennel and asparagus 55
    digestive enzyme production 11
    phyto salad 66–7
    phyto salad lunchbox 69
    smoked salmon ceviche 84
    terra mare salad with marine Phukka 88
    toasted slaw with halloumi and lemony buttermilk dressing 89
    warm lentil 87
    warm red rice with courgettes 90
salmon
    avocado and smoked salmon 46
    phyto salad lunchbox 69
    smoked salmon ceviche 84
    smoked salmon cream cheese spread 77
    salmon baked with seaweed

pesto 132
salsa
    avocado and lime 75
    salsa verde with seaweed 117
sambal, dry coconut 120
satiety 19
sauerkraut
    mushroom omelette with red sauerkraut 38
    red cabbage 185
sausage and Mediterranean veg tray bake 154
SCOBY 180
sea bass with seaweed salsa verde 135
seafood
    Brazilian-style crab 110
    crab spaghetti with seaweed 101
    Michael's mussels 98
    prawns with pasta and seaweed 138
    seafood with seaweed risotto 139
    squid Provençal 142
    terra mare salad with marine Phukka 88
    Thai prawns with coconut milk and seaweed 141
seaweed
    baked salmon with seaweed pesto 132
    crab spaghetti with seaweed 101
    dry coconut sambal 120
    green gazpacho with seaweed 63
    lemon and coriander hummus with seaweed 74
    nutrition 17, 88
    prawns with pasta and seaweed 141
    salsa verde with seaweed 117
    sea bass with seaweed salsa verde 135
    seafood with seaweed risotto 139
    seaweed miso soup 61
    sour cream and seaweed muffins 83
    Thai-flavoured seaweed crackers 79
    Thai prawns with coconut milk and seaweed 141
    tuna and veg stir-fry with seaweed 109
    turmeric spiced omelette with seaweed 38
seeds
    bircher muesli with kefir 45
    creamy pineapple smoothie 51
    flaxseed crackers 78
    healthy homemade granola 34
    mug bread 194

seeded soda bread 196
Thai-flavoured seaweed
  crackers 79
slaw, toasted with halloumi and
  lemony buttermilk dressing 89
sleep quality 20
smoked mackerel and kale
  kedgeree 47
smoked mackerel pâté 75
smoked salmon
  and avocado 46
  ceviche 84
  cream cheese spread 77
  with scrambled eggs 37
smoothies
  clever guts green 48
  creamy pineapple 51
  Dr Tim's 50
snacks 18, 201
soda bread, seeded 196
soups
  green gazpacho with seaweed
    63
  lentil and tomato 62
  pink celeriac and beetroot 64
  satiety 19
  seaweed miso 61
  vegetable bouillon 60
sour cream and seaweed muffins
  83
sourdough bread, no-knead
  198–9
spinach
  clever guts green smoothie 48
  creamy nutmeg 160
  Dr Tim's smoothie 50
  prawns with pasta and seaweed
    138
  Quorn and parsnip cottage
    pie 148
  spinach and ricotta blinis 80
  spinach dahl 112
  toasted slaw with halloumi and
    lemony buttermilk dressing
    89
  warm lentil salad 87
squid
  Provençal 142
  terra mare salad with marine
    Phukka 88
starch, resistant 40, 41, 176
steak with guacamole and
  blistered tomatoes 153
stir-fries
  green banana and pepper 163
  marinated tofu with noodles
    144
  tuna and veg with seaweed
    109
store cupboard ingredients 28–9
strawberries
  Dr Tim's smoothie 50
  strawberry chia 'jam' 208

stress 22
sugars 10, 12
sweet potatoes
  purple sweet potato and
    blackberry pie 210
sweet potato, kale and cod
  fishcakes 136
sweeteners, artificial 11

tahini drizzle 95
temptation 20
terra mare salad with marine
  Phukka 88
Thai-flavoured seaweed crackers
  79
Thai prawns with coconut milk
  and seaweed 138
thiamin 106
tofu
  Chinese noodle jar 70
  kale and tofu scramble 93
  marinated stir-fry with noodles
    144
tomatoes 24
  aubergine parmigiana 96
  Brazilian-style crab 110
  breakfast fry-up with green
    bananas 41
  crab spaghetti with seaweed
    101
  green gazpacho with seaweed
    63
  lentil and tomato soup 62
  Quorn and parsnip cottage
    pie 148
  sausage and Mediterranean veg
    tray bake 154
  slow roasted 172
  squid Provençal 142
  steak with guacamole and
    blistered tomatoes 153
  turkey and mushroom
    bolognese 131
  vegetable and paneer curry
    145
  vegetable-rich tomato sauce
    168
  warm lentil salad 87
tuna and veg stir-fry with
  seaweed 109
turkey and mushroom bolognese
  131
turmeric
  turmeric coronation chicken
    111
  dry coconut sambal 120
  nutrition 17
  onion and courgette bhajis 162
  tea 21
  turmeric buttermik dressing
    119
  turmeric spiced omelette with
    seaweed 38

variety 8
vegetables *see also specific
vegetables*
  Chinese noodle jar 70
  cruciferous 94
  Japanese-style quick pickled
    veg 167
  Mediterranean roasted, pearl
    barley and eggs 105
  nightshade family 24
  phyto salad 66–7
  quick garlic-fried greens 161
  sausage and Mediterranean veg
    tray bake 154
  variety 11, 14, 17
  vegetable and paneer curry
    145
  vegetable bouillon 60
  vegetable ferments 187
  vegetable-rich tomato sauce
    168

walnuts
  chocolate and walnut bites 202
  chocolate aubergine cake 202
  exotic carrot cake 205
  mug bread 194
water intake 19
watercress
  blood orange salad with toasted
    coriander 55
  green gazpacho with seaweed
    63
  smoked salmon ceviche 84
weight control 11, 20
willpower 20

xanthan gum 13

yoghurt 32
  beetroot and yoghurt dip 72
  with chia jam and toasted
    pistachios 35
  clever guts green smoothie 48
  coriander chicken with yoghurt
    and fennel 128
  Dr Tim's smoothie 50
  with granola and diced pear 32
  lemon and coriander hummus
    with seaweed 74
  nutrition 17
  smoked mackerel pâté 75
yuzu juice, smoked salmon
  ceviche 84